12-12-74

Good Night, Mr. Christopher

Good Night, Mr. Christopher

PATRICIA TAYLERT McIVERS

SHEED AND WARD, INC.
Subsidiary of Universal Press Syndicate
New York

Library of Congress Catalog Card Number 74-10160

ISBN: 0-8362-0592-8

To young people everywhere—
that they may see life as a precious gift
and live it to the fullest measure

Contents

SONG

What is a boy? A joy
With a lick of hair hanging in his eyes.
There's a smudge on his face
Just in case he should run into the guys.

Don't be surprised if he treasures
The thing he made in the garage on the floor—
More than he treasures the brand new toy
You bought in the Christmas store.

Supposin' he loses his baseball cap
He'll set your house on its ear . . .
But give him a problem that's a problem
And a smile will cover his fear.

What is a boy—tell me,
Is he less than a man, or more?
Well, he's wisdom, with freckles on his face . . .
A smile this old world cannot erase.
And if you're lucky, he's somethin'
To live your whole life for.

1

Another Time,
Another Place

We were sitting on the side of the hill, Vicky and I; just sitting there, feeling the dampness of the grass under us. On the opposite hill, a light twinkled on and winked at us through the early evening fog. A distant bell-tower tolled the hour. Five o'clock. "We ought to be getting on home," I said absently to the dog. But something held me. As we sat gazing at the other hill, another light blinked on, and another. Not too far off, the barking of another dog welcomed home his master. Our hill remained dark but, now, the other hill methodically began to illuminate itself, like the footlights coming on a giant stage. It reminded me of something, but I just couldn't pinpoint it. I sat there expectantly as my mind wandered back through the years, and I remembered another hill, covered with snow and laughter, and sliced and pathed by the markings of skis and toboggans carrying red-cheeked young-sters to an abrupt stop in the nearest snow bank.

Among the group of fun-seekers on our hill were three young boys. One, a little shy perhaps, cautiously tried out a gentle slope. The other two little roughnecks "belly-whacked" fearlessly over a hand-packed jump.

The hill was located in Livingston, New Jersey, the storybook town we had lived in before coming to California. I remembered it all so well now: the lovely woods and brook behind our house; that one big Christmas tree in front of the town hall each year; and the Hilltoppers drum and bugle corps, all red and gold, coming right down the middle of the main street on the Fourth of July. It was a great life for a boy!

In summertime in Livingston, our three boys played in the woods all day, wearing cowboy hats, carrying sidearms, and stalking all kinds of bad guys and big game. Chris had the red hat, and only occasionally would I see it dart from behind a bush and take cover in the shadow of a rock. Even a big guy of six years old couldn't be too careful. Kevin had the black hat, and, being Chris' senior by a comfortable margin of two years, he led the pack. Mark didn't stalk. At ten, he was above all that. I hardly saw any of them except at meals, when a couple of short blasts on Dad's old Boy Scout bugle brought them out of the thicket.

Home for us now is on the Palos Verdes

Peninsula in Southern California. We had made many business-related moves before coming to California, and though we had great hopes of loving it here, we were quite disappointed.

And Christmas in California was a real shock! After the beautiful snows, the sleigh bells and real pines of the East, we found it difficult to get used to fake decorations, Santa arriving in a camper, and Christmas shopping in Bermuda shorts. Like many families who are frequently uprooted, we made sure to carry our many traditions with us—most of ours revolving around Christmas.

Our biggest tradition surrounding Christmas was Midnight Mass. We never missed. Chris especially loved it, and hurried us out of the house much too early, to insure our getting a front seat in church. Another of our favorite traditions was watching Charles Dickens' "A Christmas Carol" on television. We watched it, together always, since the kids were barely old enough to understand, and we seemed to feel that it helped us to renew the real meaning of Christmas. I never failed to cry my eyes out when Tiny Tim died. There was just something about that scene, where the father comes in and tells his wife that he went out to the little green place where they laid the boy, and how he seemed to feel the boy slip a little hand into his, telling his Dad that he was peaceful at last. And, oh!, that empty chair by the chimney corner! The boys used to laugh at me for being so sentimental.

When summer vacation time rolled around, and

3

Dad got his annual two weeks off, we had to find something a little closer to Palos Verdes than the Adirondack Mountains (our favorite haunt in days gone by). We soon discovered Lake Arrowhead, a beautiful spot a mile high in the San Bernardino Mountains. It always reminded us a little of the East, with its scent of pines, scampering wild life, and welcome solitude surrounding the blue lake.

In spite of all our efforts, it was hard to adjust to the West Coast. Our house had come complete with carpet, drapes, landscaping and every electrical appliance known to man. It didn't need me. The children were bored, too, and immediately required a full-time chauffeur to transport them to and from school or to meet with their friends.

In Livingston, they rode horses, played football (Chris broke a collar bone three times, and Kev was always in one kind of cast or other). The two older boys won their junior lifesaving badges at the local pool. Mark was in a drum and bugle corps, and we followed them up and down the East Coast as they competed for top honors. When we moved to California, we were so determined to keep him with a corps, that, for more than a year and a half, we drove an hour each way, three times a week, on the freeways just to keep up with the Lakewood Ambassadors' practice schedule. Kev was so full of the joy of living that it seemed he had to be on six teams at one time, have a house full of hungry friends, and wring as much out of each day as life and limb would tolerate.

4

But Chris was the one, if a parent can say such a thing. He was the happy medium between the other two boys—a spunky, yet thoughtful boy with a remarkable sense of humor. Chris wasn't a practical jokester or a teller of funny stories. But he loved to laugh and to jest. He loved to give and take the jibes of his friends. He often looked for the lighter side, but really, deep down, he was a serious, purposeful boy, never far from what he thought was important and necessary to the moment or to life itself. The pompous, the verbose, the braggart were not his cup of tea. He loved nature, animals, and quiet, intelligent people. They were his source of fun. He enjoyed an hour spent joking and talking about tropical fish with his friend, Christopher Wong, or a game of chess with Dad, a pool game with Mark or Kev—all played in a spirit of good-natured fun, but yet serious and directed. Chris had a way of looking at life which cracked us up at the most unexpected times, and made any problem we encountered seem trivial. He straightened out family squabbles, planned surprises for Father's Day and organized birthdays. He wouldn't let us say a word against anyone, inside the house or out. It wasn't that he ever lectured. He just thought well of everyone. He was Christmas; he was summer vacations; he put it all together. . . .

It was quite dark now on our quiet hill, and a chill ran over me as I watched a man emerge from a truck and climb toward the place where we sat. I sat motionless, my arm around the dog, my hillside companion. The man came to within a few yards of where we were sitting.

"Better get along, Miss," he said gently. "Not safe around here after dark."

"Come, Vicki," I whispered, and dodging between the bouquets of flowers, we ran to the bottom of the hill, jumped into the car, and headed home.

2

The Long Search

Fall always seemed a sad time. I dreaded having the children go back to school...though in retrospect, I was wrong. The schools in Palos Verdes were excellent, the weather beautiful, and the children in robust good health. That particular fall of 1968 rolled along rather smoothly.

We bought the usual school supplies, the varsity band began practicing for the football season, with Mark on snare drum, and Kev made the high school basketball team. How lucky we were! But we didn't realize it.

It was the middle of October when we were awakened early one morning by Chris's screaming. Half drowsy, Bill and I ran in to him, thinking he was having a nightmare. He was sitting up in bed holding his head and screaming, "My eyes, my eyes!" If you knew Chris as we did, you'd know that he was no complainer. One time, when he was just a tyke, he was ill and had locked himself in the bathroom. On the other side of the door, frustrated and helpless, I kept begging him to let me in. I'll always remember his words, "Mom, when I have a problem I can't handle, I'll let you know." He wasn't being surly. That was just Chris—quite the master of himself and most reluctant to ask help from anyone. This morning was different. He was panic-stricken. Bill held him while I ran for the medicine cabinet. We gave him aspirin, and coaxed down a warm drink. It seemed to do the trick, and he soon went back to sleep, and we, back to bed.

He seemed fine the next morning, but I made an appointment with our family doctor. On the appointed day, after a long wait, we were admitted to the inner sanctum. The doctor went through the usual routine—tapping on the knees, looking at the tongue, in the ears, etc. The doctor asked me if there was any history of migraine headaches in our family. Well, Bill's had a few, I told him, maybe four in our twenty years of marriage. The doctor concluded that Chris was a "migraine person"—his problem was emotionally induced. Case dismissed!

About a month later Chris had the same experience, this time with more severity and accompanied by violent vomiting. Aspirin didn't seem to touch the problem this time. The previous summer, while we were on vacation, he had had a hard bout with the flu accompanied by vomiting and a pharmacist had prescribed some tranquilizing medication. Now I gave him one of the tranquilizers I had bought in the mountains, and soothed him off to sleep. As soon as he was comfortable, I got the doctor on the phone. Another appointment was made and kept, but Chris and I were disappointed since no new techniques were employed, and we came away feeling that we had wasted a couple of hours. The doctor still maintained that Chris was a hyper-nervous child, a judgment which couldn't have been further from the truth.

Nevertheless, Bill and I began looking for some "pressure situation" either at school or at home, something which might have been triggering the headaches. Open House at Ridgecrest School came about that time, and the teachers had nothing but the best to say for Chris' work and attitude.

As the days went on, I noticed that he had begun gagging on his food, and occasionally vomiting a mouthful. From all indications, it still sounded like nerves, but we could uncover no earthly reason for the abrupt change in him.

A week later, he had another violent headache, but this time he banged his head on the wall in frustration and pain, and vomited where he stood. I gave him an aspirin with a tranquilizer, for at this point the only possible way in which I could help him was to put him to sleep. As soon as he was comfortably settled in bed, I raced for the phone and called the same doctor. When I tried, half crying, to explain that Chris wouldn't vomit on the carpet unless he was really in trouble, the doctor actually yelled at me, "It's a psychiatric problem. Get him to a good psychiatrist and keep him there!" He hung up. I put my head down on the kitchen sink and cried. Then I went back up to Chris.

I have often wondered about some of these medical men who like to play God. We met so many of them, especially the fifty-dollar-a-visit variety. On many occasions, I had to take Chris out of school, neglect other duties, wait in their assorted offices for at least an hour, only to come away with the feeling of disgust at their condescending attitudes, their patronizing smiles. One has to wonder if it has ever occurred to them that many of us mothers have as much education as they. We are closer to the problem than they could ever be. And, being better acquainted with the history and personality of the child, could provide a valuable source of information leading to a correct diagnosis, if only they would listen. Instead, we hear the same old clichés, in office after office. "I'm sure it's nothing to worry about." "Is there something wrong with the home atmosphere?" "I wouldn't let it bother me if I were you." No, they probably wouldn't—not unless it were their child who was suffering. I was very bitter on this subject. We contacted some fifteen specialists, yet it took two years of agony for Chris and the whole family before we could find one man who would take a genuine interest in the case.

With no other route to go, we took our family

doctor's advice and secured the services of one of the very best psychiatrists in the area, Dr. Alberta Samuelson. She was a brilliant woman with a large following. She talked to Chris and me together, with Chris separately, and finally, with Dad. Her conclusion was that she found no psychiatric basis for Chris' problems. We were grateful, but we were right back where we had started, and Chris was getting worse all the time.

Our relatives and neighbors were becoming interested in Chris' problems and were offering all kinds of suggestions, for which we were grateful. In November, 1968, someone told us about an excellent gastro-neurologist in the Redondo Beach area. I made an appointment for the next week, and once more lost a couple of hours between the waiting room and the "family history." We made another appointment for a complete G.I. series, no fun for a young boy. This was completed a week later in the doctor's offices. The result: negative.

Meanwhile, Chris was losing weight and missing more and more school. He was in intermediate school, seventh grade, and constantly embarrassing himself by getting sick in front of his friends. By Christmas, there was hardly a day when he didn't go to school with a headache and upset stomach. When the phone rang during the day, I always knew it was the school nurse calling me to pick him up. I often wondered what the school personnel thought of us. They didn't know at that time that I used to drop Chris off in the

morning and cry all the way home. I never left the
house, because I knew that he'd never make it
through the day. However, we were still being
advised by all his doctors to keep him in school, for
fear of building psychological problems. I'll always
remember one day when the nurse called me
during the lunch hour. As Chris came out of school,
looking sick enough to die, a group of girls standing
near the car shouted, "Weirdo!" I could have cried,
but didn't dare.

Over and over, I renewed my promise to him to
get to the bottom of the problem, and Chris, true to
his spunky nature, never gave up trying. He still
rode his skate-board, played basketball, and put up
a great front for the neighborhood kids. But things
were getting rough at home. Bills were mounting
up, nerves were taut. The other boys found it
difficult to concentrate on homework and exams. I
began checking out nutrition books from the library, and spent a good deal of time buying and
cooking health foods. At the dinner table, no one
could raise a fork without stealing a glance at
Chris, to determine whether or not his dinner was
going to stay down. It rarely did. But the problem
was so erratic! We had seen him run for the
bathroom and vomit violently, then come back to
the table and, I'm sure, for no other reason than to
reassure us, pick up his fork and eat a full meal.
For some unexplained reason it always stayed
down the second time.

We were getting little sleep; we lay awake long

hours, talking and trying to come up with some logical explanation for Chris' illness. Exhaustion and worry were certainly taking their toll on our once happy home. One terrible night, Dad came home particularly tired. Mark and Kev were in the middle of January '69 exams. Chris was sicker than usual that night, and curled up in a big overstuffed chair in our bedroom. He looked terrible. I started to say something to Dad about doing something for the boy, and poor Dad, exhausted and worried about mounting medical bills, shouted, "Don't take that kid to another damn doctor!" Chris crumbled and the tears streamed down his cheeks. Later that night, in bed, Bill tried to reason with me. There was nothing wrong with Chris' heart, lungs, digestive tract, coordination, or with his psyche, he pointed out. "Believe the doctors," he begged, "before you put us all in the poorhouse!" That night, I think I felt sicker than Chris. Now, no one would listen, not even Dad. But the thing that kept nagging me was that I knew Chris. He wasn't a complainer, a school-hater, an attention-seeker. I watched him like a hawk, the black circles under his eyes when he slept. I began keeping charts on everything he did, everything he ate. But there just wasn't any pattern.

Chris had always had a very light hay-fever condition and when someone suggested that this whole problem might be caused by allergy, we contacted a reputable allergist in our area. Each time we tried a new doctor, we had renewed hope.

On the way to the allergist we stopped at a Seven-Eleven Store for a "slurpy," a snow-cone topped with flavored syrup, and about the only thing he could keep down for sure. The allergist was a tall, skeleton of a man, obviously a nervous wreck himself. During the office consultation, he told us of his only son, a migraine person, who had such a great mind that he, as a father, could not allow it to go to waste. So he kept the boy in law school, but only with the support of a psychiatrist whom the boy visited three times a week. After an hour visit, during which he did most of the talking, he decided that Chris must be the same type of person as his son. Chris and I kept exchanging glances. Since we had no other logical route to follow, Chris went through the allergy tests, which revealed that he might have a very mild allergy to grasses or weeds. He began the series of shots on a three-times-a-week basis, though I think we both knew it was fruitless.

It was about this time, that we chanced to meet a wonderful man—Joaquin Acosta, then assistant to the chancellor, at U.C.L.A. By now, Bill and I were so distraught that Chris was the first thing on our lips. This very kind gentleman spoke to us about U.C.L.A. Medical Center, its brilliant staff and research facilities. He encouraged us to take Chris there and promised his support in putting us in touch with the best medical people available. We left him, remembering that, if ever we should need him, we had only to pick up the phone. As stupid as it may sound, I know I had heard somewhere that medical centers were big, bare, impersonal places where persons might be treated as guinea pigs, so we were reluctant to try it. Besides, we had within a radius of a few miles the very best medical men in all fields.

The allergy shots yielded nothing. The nurse in that office, however, suggested that Chris' post-nasal drip could contribute to his stomach problems and suggested we try an ear, nose, and throat specialist. We followed through on this suggestion, but again, it was not the answer. This doctor, however, was alarmed enough about Chris' condition to take me aside and suggest that if it were his boy, he'd get him to a good neurosurgeon at once. The thought frightened me, and yet, I couldn't believe that I hadn't come up with that idea myself.

We were referred to a doctor in Redondo Beach, a man whose reputation was supported by two close friends of ours, one of whom credited him with having saved her husband's life. On the first visit he put Chris through the usual series of tests, i.e., touching finger to nose, standing on one leg, or with one foot directly in front of the other to test balance, etc. I never imagined that in years to come, I would catch Chris testing himself time and again in just that manner. The doctor found the boy to be very sound, but just to be certain, he sent him to Little Company of Mary Hospital in Torrance, for a brain wave test, brain scan and X-rays. When I called a couple of days later for the results, I was

15

told to take Chris out of school and bring him in. We were both certain that the tests had brought something to light, but we were wrong. After a few spins in his swivel chair, and a prolonged, "W-E-L-L," during which time my heart sank a mile, he said that the tests were completely negative. I walked out of that office on cloud nine, but Chris was despondent. He knew that he was sick, desperately sick. For him, it meant going back to school feeling "lousy," and trying to convince his friends and family that his ills were not psychosomatic. I asked, "How about a slurpy?" His answer: "Forget it."

We finished out the spring somehow, and Chris did exceptionally well on his June exams. He tried out for the Majors in the Little League, but failed to make it. He was just too weak to put his best effort into it. We went back to Arrowhead that summer of 1969 but it was no fun. He was sick the whole time.

Fall of the same year found Chris in the eighth grade—his last year in Ridgecrest Intermediate School. He was too sick to make the first day, or the second, or the third. Over everyone's objections, we made another appointment with the neurosurgeon and again Chris went into the hospital for all the tests. After two whole days of careful testing, we drew another blank. In pure desperation, we contacted the psychiatrist and she took him into her class of four children, as she put it, strictly by default. It yielded nothing, and again she released him.

Meanwhile, that wonderful kid was still

hanging in there both with his friends and with his eighth-grade studies. He was falling a bit behind, though, and insisted on staying up half the night trying to catch up with the class. He had always been such a good student, and now that he was missing days he found it a tremendous effort to stay with the class. Every night I'd watch his frail frame hunched over the desk. He was trying so hard. He was feeling so badly. At this point he was vomiting three times a day and suffering from constant headaches. He was on so many different kinds of medications that he was listless all of the time, and spent most of his at-home time just lying on the couch. And I couldn't help him.

I had noticed a slight curvature of the spine and thought, just perhaps, this could be affecting his nervous system in some way. We consulted a chiropractor (whom I picked out of the yellow pages of the phone book). By this time I was "running scared." I didn't know where to turn. Along with the vomiting, Chris had always complained of a lot of pain in the back of his neck. The chiropractor found a pinched nerve in that area, and again, we had hope. We visited his office for adjustments twice a week for a couple of months, and for a time, I thought Chris perked up a little. But it didn't last and we gave it up.

He was getting steadily worse, now adding another symptom to the list. He complained of seeing double. I experienced a terrible shock one morning while sitting on his bed; when I got eyeball to eyeball with him, I could actually see his eyes "jigging" in his head in time with his pulse beat. That first night when he shouted, "My eyes, my eyes," came slamming back at me. Immediately, I picked up the phone and made an appointment with an ophthalmologist. I was sure we had hit upon something this time. After a thorough examination, and the use of a lot of medical terms, he did write a prescription for glasses.

Chris just couldn't wait until they were ready. What a simple solution to his long-endured illness! Finally we got the call and went down to pick up the glasses. Chris was more eager than ever to stay up with his books that night. As the days went on, he tried to think positively, but the headaches and the vomiting continued.

By now, his main source of nutrition came out of the blender. I concocted mixtures rich enough in vitamins and protein to sustain the Los Angeles Rams. To give the impression, however, that he lived on a bunch of mushy health foods and milkshakes would be erroneous. Like all boys, Chris had his favorite foods: lobster dripping with drawn butter, shrimp, tacos, strawberries, roast beef, cherries (with stems), walnuts and cheesecake headed the list. Quite frequently, he would astonish us by putting away two tacos and a strawberry shortcake in one sitting. One peculiarity about his eating was that he always knew whether or not a meal was going to stay down. Either it stayed in a lump in his chest, or, as he described it, a valve just to the right of center, where the esophagus meets the stomach, would open. His face would relax, and we'd know that it was going to be O.K. To see him enjoy a meal seemed to be the first thing on all of our minds. He was never nauseous, and, being an active kid, and right in the middle of his teen-age growing period, he was always starved. This made it all the more difficult for all of us. Everything in the supermarket looked good to him. Everything on a restaurant menu was enticing. He always ate with great gusto, and then there would be that awful few minutes in the bathroom, and he'd come away looking drained and discouraged. It depressed us all to watch him, and there was no doubt that our days were made or broken by the moods of his erratic stomach. Dad called from work every day to inquire about him, and the other boys came home from school, poor kids, looking as though they were afraid to ask, "How's the little 'Creep'?" Over the years, "Creep" had replaced Chris, but I assure you it was a term most affectionately used. After all, he was the little brother.

As Christmas, 1969, approached, things were looking bleak. For some reason, "Papilledema," a term the ophthalmologist had mentioned, stuck in my mind. From time to time, I still consulted the psychiatrist on the phone, not only to help us to handle Chris, but also to help keep our family ties intact and preserve sanity. She was wonderfully generous with sound advice and encouragement. During one of our conversations, I casually mentioned the term "Papilledema," and she picked it up at once. Being careful not to alarm me, she said the condition usually indicates pressure on the brain and encouraged me to get Chris back to the neurosurgeon at once. We made another appointment, and again poor Chris landed back in the hospital. One of his big traumas was having that plastic bracelet clipped onto his wrist. He often referred to this procedure as "being plugged into the hospital." On many a later visit, when he found himself dropping into various hospitals for this test or that, he made a joke of walking down the exact center of the hall on the way to the lab. He used to kid me and say that if he walked too close to the doors, a long arm would reach out and slap on the bracelet—trapped!

This trip to the hospital found him going through the same brain-scan, X-rays, etc. Our follow-up visit to the neurosurgeon's office fell on December 23, 1969—the day before our beloved Christmas Eve. The kids were already out of school for the holidays, hence a bit of pressure was lifted. Nevertheless, I shook so hard on the way that I could hardly drive the car. Chris kept up his endless comical chatter, trying to bolster my spirits, and I bantered back, talking too much and laughing too loudly.

There was a Christmas tree in the waiting room this time, and as I sat there, my mind was spinning with last-minute preparations for the big holiday. I remember thinking that Christmas would either come joyfully as usual, or it would never come again, depending on what we were about to hear. The nurse called our name, and we were again ushered into the semiplush office which had become so familiar to us. The doctor was sitting in his big swivel chair, hands clasped as if in prayer, an open folder on the desk before him. "Chris," he began, "how are you doing?" I glanced at Chris. A smile spread from ear to ear. "Great," he said in a bold voice. "Just fine." It always came out sounding like "Foin." "What a kid," I thought. I just couldn't believe his poise. His face betrayed no sign of anxiety at all. Without another word, the doctor swung his chair over to me, right up close, knee to knee. He placed his hands on my shoulders and shook me just a little. "Mother," he asked, "when are you going to believe that there's nothing wrong with this boy?" I felt at once like a dumb little kid and a beaten woman. I was worried about Chris' reaction, since by this time we were almost hoping they would find something so that we could zero in on the problem. I remember driving home after the previous visit to the doctor. Chris had been so "down." But this time, whether he had been so worried and now was relieved, or whether it was the fact that the holiday season was upon us, he was exuberant. When we got into the car, I said, "Merry Christmas, Honey." His answer: "How about a slurpy?" He had two—grape!

Christmas that 1969 was great. We watched Dickens, went to Midnight Mass, ate homemade cookies, decorated to the hilt, opened presents, and cooked Christmas dinner. It was some dinner— everything the budget would allow, and a lot more. But no one ate it. Chris was sick as usual, but after a half-hour snooze, he was up and away again, his great little spirit not wanting to miss a single moment of that wonderful day. Twilight meant time to build a fire in the fireplace, turn on the outside lights, and put the old standards on the phonograph. It wasn't long before Bing Crosby's "White Christmas" swept away our troubles and once again molded us into one happy family.

January passed without incident. Mark and Kevin wore their new shirts and pants back to school and began the big push toward midterm exams. Chris continued in the same pattern—sick most of the time—but with the late-night home-work and great effort keeping up with the class. He did his usual thing on exams—almost straight A's. We just couldn't believe it!

Just as the weight of exams lifted, we received word that Grandma and Grandpa were coming out from Rochester, New York, for a prolonged stay. It was just the shot in the arm we all needed. I had written them for almost two years about Chris and Grandpa was very concerned about the "little Creep." It was great fun making preparations for their arrival—moving beds, moving kids, cleaning out closets. We all met them at the airport and Grandpa took me aside and told me that Chris looked pretty good to him, though a lot taller and lankier than when he had last seen him. Grandpa chalked this up to puberty and a growing streak.

We had dinner at our house that night, and cocktails before dinner in the backyard. While we enjoyed our drinks, Chris and Kevin played basketball on our little court, and for a few minutes, I felt almost guilty to have alarmed my dad. Chris was full of vinegar and amused us by trying to out-shoot Kev, who was six feet tall and nearly a hundred pounds heavier than Chris. Chris' pride contributed to his cleverness, and for a month or so, he never seemed to be sick when anyone was watching. But I was watching him, and things went from bad to worse.

One evening when I was preparing dinner, I received a phone call from the mother of one of Chris' friends. She sounded upset. She began to unravel a story of how Chris had fallen into the bushes at school that day, incoherent, and not able to recognize his friends. Her son, Mike, who was in the same class with Chris, got to him first, and apparently what he saw scared him to death. A moment or two later the vice-principal came out and carried Chris into the nurse's office, where he rested until he regained himself. I was never informed of any of this by the school authorities. When I confronted Chris with the story, he made light of it and said that he had just lost his balance. I called Chris' friend, Mike, and he was almost in tears while telling me the details. I knew Mike and I believed him. I realized now that Chris was going through more—much more—than even we realized. "Dear God," I begged, "please help me." Here was a boy only fourteen years old, suffering terribly, perhaps even dying, and now, trying to shield the worst of it from his parents. During the endless hours of that sleepless night I decided it was all up to me. I didn't care who complained and I didn't care what it cost—I had to make a move.

My fingers could hardly dial the number of the U.C.L.A. chancellor's office. Having been turned off so many times, I was dumbfounded when Joaquin Acosta, the good man we had spoken with at church, came to the phone immediately. He asked me only one question, "Is this the same boy you talked to me about nearly a year ago?" In spite of all of our efforts in the interim, I felt like an unconcerned parent saying, "Yes." He told me to hang up the phone and to stay right there. Within three minutes, I received a call from a Dr. John Menkes, at the Marion Davies Children's Clinic at U.C.L.A. Medical Center. I fully expected him to say, "Bring Chris in a week from Thursday." Instead, he said, "Be here at 1:00 P.M. tomorrow."

The Marion Davies Clinic was a complete and pleasant surprise. The waiting room was large and cheerful. Glass walls revealed rolling lawns, flowering trees, and tropical plants. The waiting room itself was colorful and incorporated just about every toy, book, picture, and accessory that could tempt a child's imagination. Most of the children around us were quite young, and I was afraid for a moment that we had come to the wrong place. But very shortly our name was called, and I found that, not only were we expected, but that they had already taken time to gather the bulk of Chris' case history. When Dr. Menkes came into the examining room I had a feeling of immediate trust. He was a kind man, with soft dark eyes, his bearded features reflecting great gentleness. He put Chris through the simplest of neurological tests and asked very few questions. While Chris was getting dressed, Dr. Menkes took me aside. I felt embarrassed. I guess I had lost confidence in myself, both as a mother and as a person. I blurted out, "My husband doesn't think Chris has a problem, but I do." In the quietest of voices, he said, simply, "I do, too. You are a very brave woman."

He told me of his suspicion—that Chris might have a brain tumor—and that he wanted Chris admitted to the hospital immediately. I suggested that Chris had had a very unpleasant experience many years before in a children's ward and asked that he be admitted to the adult section. Chris was then fourteen years old. The good doctor agreed without an argument, and directed us to the admitting office.

There was no wait there, and Chris and I were impressed with the friendliness of everyone we met. They weren't saying, "See a psychiatrist." They were saying, "We believe you." We signed a few short papers, admitting him the next morning. Then we returned home to pick up pajamas and a

25

few necessities.

Dad and the boys were shocked when we told them the news. The next morning Dad stayed home from work, and the three of us drove back to U.C.L.A.—Bill, Chris and I—and a little brown suitcase.

3

God Said, "No!"

The admitting office was empty, save for the very pleasant woman we had encountered the night before. Bill paced up and down the hall while she guided us through the barest mimimum of procedures—always conveying the feeling that "you're going to like it here."

Instead of our being wrenched away from Chris, as is the case in most hospitals, we were invited to accompany him to his room—a four-bed male suite in the Neuropsychiatric Institute. It was a lovely room with a wall of picture windows overlooking the beautiful U.C.L.A. campus. We could see Chris' relief when asked to drop into a little private bath and change into his own pajamas. How he hated those hospital gowns! Just as soon as he was settled in bed, a nurse came around and told him he could order anything he wanted—ice cream, soft drinks, jello, etc. She brought a menu both for the evening meal and for breakfast the following morning. Looking at him there in his new pajamas, making instant friends of the other three men in the room, my heart, instead of being light, felt like lead with the thought of what might be in store for him.

The next week and a half was trying, to say the very least. We spent every day—all day—at the hospital. There were questions to be asked, more case histories to be collected, and dozens of difficult tests for Chris. Many of his young friends drove that hour on the freeway to see him, as did Grandpa, Grandma, and our very special friends from Santa Monica, with whom my Dad and Mom now resided. Chris made a very special friend of the nice man in the bed next to him. The man had some sort of eye problem and Chris worried much more about him than he did about himself. Although the man spoke very little English, there was an instant rapport between them, and quite a mutual interest in the game of chess. From several paces down the hall, we could hear a hearty whoop and a holler every time a knight was captured, or a king put in check.

We spent a lot of time in that hall just out of earshot of the occupants of the room. There were several doctors on the case, the chief surgeon being Dr. Paul Crandall, whom we had not met at this point. Many times a day we would get the "high sign" to step out into the hall and hear the results of one test or another.

About the second day there, through the medium of more brain scans, they had located the tumor. The subsequent tests, which lasted for almost two weeks, were to determine the exact position and extent of the growth before surgery. I will never forget the day they found it. Dr. Menkes was now more or less off the case, since Chris was out of his Pediatric Department, but he met us in the hall that day and, looking on the verge of tears, gave us the news. He explained that there are several types of tumors, and they were hoping this to be a liquid variety, which might be drained first, and then removed. We asked him if it was big, and he said, "Yes." "How big?" we wanted to know. He couldn't say it. "Bigger than a grape?" I ventured. "Yes," was all he could manage. His eyes were scanning the floor. "As big as a golf ball?" I tried again. My head was swimming. He was suffering, too, I knew, and I felt both sad and gratified to know that such a great man possessed such a big heart. Finally, with great difficulty, he whispered, "About the size of a baseball."

Impossible! When I thought of that dear head with the brown hair and the infectious smile—his whole head wasn't much bigger than that! Through the haze, I tried to reason that certainly a thing of that proportion would have affected his mind or his coordination. Oh! No, God, please. I looked from the doctor's face to Bill's and back again. They looked like stone. I was crying . . . half out of my mind when I left Bill and the doctor standing in the hall.

29

I was angry, too, mad as hell as I ran down three flights of stairs to the lobby and put a dime in a pay phone. I dialed the Redondo Beach number of the neurosurgeon. The nurse's voice said he couldn't be disturbed. I don't remember what I said, but in about ten seconds he was on the other end of the line. "We're at U.C.L.A. Medical Center," I blurted. "They found a tumor as big as a baseball." The words that came back hit me like a bolt of lightning: "That's what I was afraid of. Have them send me a written report." He hung up. His words of December 23—just a couple of months before— came slamming back at me: "Mother, when are you going to believe there's nothing wrong with this boy?" Dear Lord, was I going mad? I must have cried out loud, because a strange man knocked on the door of the phone booth and asked me if he could help.

Bill, Dear Bill, was standing in the hall alone when I came back upstairs. No decision was made, not a word passed between us. We just went into Chris' room, and as if of one mind . . . told him that they had found a little tumor, a liquid one the size of a grape, and that they were sure—we lied with a smile—that they could drain and remove it with no difficulty at all.

Chris had some really frightening tests to go through, some so dangerous that we had to sign a form giving our consent. The angiogram, when they put a needle into the groin and inject dye into the bloodstream, and the pneumoencephalogram, when

30

air is pumped into the cranium, while the patient is strapped into a chair and spun around, both terrified me. I had heard they were both frightening and painful and begged the doctors to anesthetize Chris first. They explained that they couldn't, but would do their best to make him groggy, thereby keeping him comfortable. Each time we signed, I made them promise to wait until we arrived in the morning before starting the test, so we could, at least, walk Chris down to the testing room. One morning we arrived to find his bed empty. The day before we had signed for the pneumoencephalogram. I was terrified—they had already taken him downstairs. I suppose we were making nuisances of ourselves, but over the past two years we had become so disenchanted with the doctors and hospitals that we just wanted to follow Chris every step of the way. Besides, now, we had a terrible secret to protect. He was a bright kid, and had ears like a fox. We were so afraid he'd overhear something of the magnitude of the surgery he was about to undergo.

The whole family then, on this particular morning, hurried down to the basement testing rooms. The basement was a maze of concrete halls with a hundred identical doors—some mysteriously closed and some standing ajar to reveal a variety of huge, forbidding machinery. Kevin zeroed in on Chris' room almost at once, and slipped out of sight into an antechamber adjoining the testing room. Through the small window in a heavy door, he saw his brother hanging upside-down in a chair and screaming. The doctor was saying, "Just one more time...just one more time." When Kev gave us a report on this, we collapsed. We waited miserably until they wheeled a sleeping, perspired, and exhausted little Chris back to his room. He slept most of the day, and when he awoke he claimed that he remembered very little of the experience.

The second week found Chris' brothers and friends on spring vacation, so they were able to spend a great deal of time visiting the hospital. We used to go up in the morning laden with collages, posters, cards, and gifts which had been laid on our doorstep by neighbors and school chums. His room at the hospital was so crammed with teen-type "junk" that you couldn't find an inch of wall showing. He had a transistor radio with earphones, and his little foot never missed a beat, tapping away under the white sheets. I used to kid him about having a tic.

The hospital food was great, according to Chris. In the two weeks before the operation, and the six after it, I don't believe he vomited once. While some of the other patients were complaining about the fare, Chris was eating like a horse! "Slow down!" I used to kid. "For the sake of your old Mom, maybe you could send a little back to the kitchen once in a while! How do you expect me to convince the doctors you've been sick for two years?" But he always countered with, "Now wait, Mom. Did it ever occur to you that it might not be my stomach, but the fault of the cook?" We had a lot of fun over this, but he knew full well how delighted we all were to see him wolf down a meal, from soup to dessert. He looked great, too. He was cheerful and gaining weight. We were exhausted and losing it.

We still hadn't met the head surgeon, an unbelievably busy man, though we kept an almost constant eye on his office door just down the hall. One afternoon I happened to be alone with Chris. Bill had gone down to the hospital business office to work out expenses, insurance, etc., when a nurse tapped me on the shoulder and told me that Dr. Crandall would see us right away. I was afraid that if I passed up the opportunity to talk with him, it might be a long wait for another. By this time, most of my courage had left me and I dreaded the encounter without Bill's being there. Dr. Paul Crandall, a tall slim man with masked expression, gave no hint of his feelings. He was completely clinical in his approach, and began saying, "I don't mind telling you that we are facing a giant of an operation." He mentioned that if all went well the operation would take from eight to ten hours, the tumor, hopefully, would be removed and since it was in the area of the medulla, we might expect that Chris would experience some problems with his coordination later on. If things did not go well, the operation would take only about five hours. He explained the procedure they followed if the tumor was malignant and couldn't be removed. An intravenous "shunt" would be introduced into the skull.

The shunt, running down behind his ear would empty into a vein in his chest, thereby relieving pressure on the brain, and making Chris more comfortable for the time he may have left.

It is a puzzle to me the way in which one's mind works at a time like this, but as exhausted as I was, and paralyzed with fear, I looked at this brilliant man and felt compassion for him. As I left his office, all I could think of to say was, "I'll pray for you." I was shaking so violently from head to foot that I had to sit down on a bench in the hall to keep my legs from buckling. I explained the procedures to Bill, and we waited several days more. The more I observed Chris in the hospital, the more I was truly convinced that there could be no malignancy. He looked so rosy, seemed so happy, and, for the first time in two years, was beginning to fill out and approach the weight a healthy fourteen-year-old should carry.

Finally, after many postponements, the operation was scheduled for Good Friday, 1970. Somehow, in spite of my great hopes, the thought went through my head, "This day, thou shalt be with me in paradise." It could mean two things. Perhaps the operation would be a complete success—that would be paradise for sure. Or perhaps the enormity of the ordeal would be more than our dear little friend could endure. Then, paradise for one of us and hell for the rest.

Driving home on the freeway Wednesday night, with our two lanky sons in the back seat, I felt it proper to summarize the situation and prepare ourselves for the two toughest days of our lives. "The best that can happen, of course, " I began, "is that Chris will come through with flying colors. The second best thing is that he dies on the operating table, and the worst is that it turns out to be malignant and he comes home to die." Bill, looking as haggard as ever I've seen a man, said, "Pat, for God's sake!" No one uttered another word the rest of the way home. There was no sleep for any of us that night. We kept meeting each other in the kitchen, crying, while putting on the teapot or sipping a glass of wine. At least an eternity passed before we saw the daylight and were on the road to U.C.L.A. again.

It was now Holy Thursday—and through the haze it dawned on me that I had not made any preparations for the last rites of our church. The nurses gave me the number of the nearest Catholic Church and a priest showed up at the hospital almost immediately. I tried to make arrangements for the Sacrament to be administered the following morning, but told the priest of my great anxieties about frightening Chris, who at this point still believed that he was to have a one-hour operation amounting to little more than a tonsillectomy. The good Lord was with us this time for just at that moment they wheeled Chris back from another test, and he was out like a light. The priest assured me he'd give Chris the short form of the Sacrament for the dying. Our darling boy never knew that, from that time on, he had one foot in heaven.

Chris was happy all that day, though apprehensive about having his head shaved. We tried to kid him about getting a "rug," setting a new fad among his peers. For the most part, though, we kept reminding him that within twenty-four hours he'd be back in his room, with all of his problems behind him, and that his hair would be back in a short month.

I asked the nurses if there was any possibility of my staying overnight with Chris. Without a moment's hesitation, they made me feel as welcome as could be imagined. I would have been willing to sit up all night in the hall—but they wouldn't hear of it. They moved his bed down the hall to a semiprivate room that would accommodate both of us. Our dear relatives from Santa Monica ran out and bought me a toothbrush and a pair of pajamas.

The operation was originally scheduled for 8:00 A.M., and the night before, Bill and the boys reluctantly took their leave, promising to be back before Chris left the floor next morning. There was little or no sleep for either Chris or me that night. Someone had brought me a little bottle of Holy Water from the Shrine at Lourdes, and each time the boy dozed off, I sprinkled it on his head and pillow.

At the crack of dawn, a pretty nurse came in and gave him a partial haircut and shampoo. Chris' tremendous sense of humor never left him, and he kept up a steady chatter which kept both the nurse and me laughing all the time. Shortly after, another nurse entered with a pan of water and all the shaving equipment. Chris made jokes about going to the electric chair. He suggested that having no hair on his head would make his black fuzz of a mustache stand out all the more. Bill and the other boys came in just as his head was being disinfected, and the tan knitted hospital cap was stretched into place.

Of course, we felt that our case was unique and about the most important thing the hospital had to deal with. But apparently we were mistaken, for Chris' operation was postponed until eleven o'clock. We had a difficult time in those few hours, making light conversation and keeping up spirits. About ten-thirty, he was sent for, and we all walked down to the operating room with him. As our pathetic procession entered the hall, I caught a glimpse of the priest I had met the night before. He was dressed in street clothes, and, as we passed, he gave a silent blessing. I guess you could say that my faith failed me right then, for I had the distinct feeling, just as Chris had kidded, that someone was going to the gallows. We followed him to the basement and right up to the double doors, above which a sign read: "POSITIVELY NO ADMITTANCE—HOSPITAL PERSONNEL ONLY." Lightly, four smiling faces kissed him goodbye, and we all said, "See you in an hour!" When the doors closed behind him, we all fell together in one melting lump of desperation.

We went back to his room, where all of his things had been. Already, in those short moments, his personal belongings had been moved around the corner to the postsurgical hall, and into a private room directly opposite the intensive care unit. We were asked to wait in the main lobby downstairs, which, of course, we did. Here, I am sure, we experienced the second longest Good Friday in history.

It was a big lobby, cool and bright, with a number of couches, chairs, and the usual potted plants. A very busy and efficient nurse occupied the desk and switchboard in one corner. After a couple of hours' wait, we were trying to talk each other into a short trip to the cafeteria for a bite to eat—but none of us would even consider it. Grandpa and Grandma came in after a while, Grandpa toting a big brown paper bag of Easter eggs which he had colored himself—and a first aid flask containing a bit of whiskey. They sat with us for quite a time, encouraging us to have a nip or to go out for lunch, but neither was appealing or seemed appropriate. I was saying the rosary—I must have said twenty of them. I kept going over the joyful mysteries because I wanted to think optimistically. From time to time, a nurse would come by and lay a hand on our shoulders, agreeing that this was the most difficult time to bear, and giving us words of encouragement.

The switchboard in the corner was busy constantly, and we kept alert for the mention of any doctor's name who was even remotely connected with the case.

At a quarter to five, I had to visit the ladies' room, which was no more than ten steps from where we were sitting. I was so "uptight" that I could not have been gone for more than three minutes at the outside. Yet, when I came out, Bill said a nurse from upstairs had come down and told him that Chris would be back in his room in half an hour. My heart stopped! "God Almighty," I thought. "No." Grandpa and Grandma had left and I remember wishing with all my heart that they were there. "Are you sure that's what she said?" I kept asking Bill. "Oh, God! It looks bad." No sooner had the words left my lips than the switchboard nurse gave us the message that Dr. Crandall wanted to meet with us in the third-floor conference room immediately. The verdict was in. I knew it! None of us, I am sure, remember the ride up on the elevator.

When the elevator door opened, the conference room was directly in front of us—door open—and Dr. Crandall, in an impeccably white coat, was waiting for us. As we passed through the door, I asked, "It's not good, is it?" His answer was that he had good news and bad. We took our positions around the conference table and the doctor began. "Well, he came through the operation in fine style ... but that tumor was malignant." I am not at all ashamed to say that the four of us sprawled over the conference table and sobbed.

There is a puzzling facet to the human spirit. You can know a thing to be true—absolutely certain, as we did when we walked through that door, but the full impact doesn't hit you—the last shred of hope doesn't leave you until the fact is put into words. We experienced this ourselves at this moment, and it became one of the deciding factors in our unanimous decision never to tell Chris the truth. When hope is gone, the natural tendency to fight goes with it—perhaps even the will to live vanishes.

The doctor was explaining his findings, and through the haze of broken minds and spirits we heard . . . "took a frozen cube . . . biopsy . . . too extensive even to touch . . . medulla blastoma . . . intravenous shunt to relieve the pressure." At one point I lifted my head from the table and shouted at the doctor, "My God, I wish you had slipped." How could we tell Chris or not tell him? How on earth could we live with this awful knowledge right down to the time when we had to watch him die? Oh, my God, how could we ever live without him!

Meanwhile, Kevin had partially recovered and was throwing questions at the doctor. "Don't you know of something, someone, perhaps in Europe . . . some new treatment?" All the time the doctor kept shaking his head and repeating the phrase, "No hope . . . no hope." He went on to say that Chris had no chance to live the normal life span. We began to rally a little and Bill asked how long Chris had to live. "About two years," was the answer. "How will he die?" I asked. His answer was just a trifle reassuring. "These people usually just sleep away."

As we walked out of that room, I recall having the feeling that I didn't know where to turn. I mean literally—right or left, up or down. But just as we stood there bewildered, the elevator door opened and Chris was wheeled off. His head was enlarged by a mountain of gauze and bandages. Both his eyes were black down to his chin. Only that little black fuzz of a mustache told us it really was our little boy. We kissed him and talked to him, though he could not hear. Then we watched numbly as they wheeled him off to intensive care.

We needed someone. I put in a call to Grandpa, who was staying with our relatives in Santa Monica. The whole clan was there within minutes. When they came we were in the lobby again. We had decided—thoughtfully—not to tell Chris the whole truth. But my dad did not agree with us. "Dad," I pleaded, "How can I face this pathetic young boy—Little League player, skate-board champion, the kid who loved life more than any of us—and say, 'Look, Honey, you have brain cancer'?" Also, consider that we had been told he would have two years to live. We knew that he could never have another happy Christmas, another carefree trip to Disneyland, or another lovely summer at Lake Arrowhead, if he knew. So we stuck to our guns and determined to keep the secret as long as we could. The doctors, too, put us under a lot of pressure. Most of them felt we were making the wrong decision. I began thinking that maybe we were taking too much upon ourselves, so a few days later, I called Chris' psychiatrist for her opinion. She put it this way: "You are four healthy people. He is one sick child. You are much more able to bear the burden of this thing than he is."

When we arrived home that Good Friday night, determined to keep our secret, one of our good neighbors followed us into the house. "You look terrible," she told me. I passed it off as having had no sleep the night before. On Saturday morning early, another wonderful neighbor (not of our faith) called and said, "I can tell by your voice that everything is all right. I just knew it would turn out well on your Good Friday." I loved her for the thought, but I could have cried.

While Chris was in intensive care, we could see him ten minutes out of every hour. He looked bad, hooked up with so many tubes to so many machines, but he was always in excellent spirits. On Sunday morning after the operation, I suddenly remembered it was Easter, and we had no baskets or gifts. Bill and I found a candy shop near home and bought a whole lot of Easter goodies. When we brought them up to Chris, I remember he said two things: "Dad, I'm sorry to spoil your Easter," and "Mom, you look terrible."

When we got home that Easter night we each had our own way of dealing with our sorrow. I usually had a highball on the kitchen bar, while I answered dozens of phone calls from concerned neighbors. Bill went to bed and read a little and thought a lot. He was trying to keep up with his job as well as running to the hospital every day; I'll never know how he did it. Mark and Kev shut themselves up in their rooms and came to grips with life and death much before their times. That particular night, I decided that if we were going to keep up this façade I should at least set my hair. So, in order not to disturb anyone, I took all the paraphernalia downstairs into the bathroom. There is a television set in the rumpus room adjoining the bathroom, and after setting a curler or two, I felt an uncontrollable urge to turn on the TV. I walked out and stood before it, then thought: "What am I doing here?" Television was the last thing on my mind. I went back to the hairsetting. A second time, I found myself standing before the television, almost without realizing it. Anger, and then fear welled up in me and I forced myself back to the task at hand. After a few more curlers, I again found myself in front of the TV. Defeated, I punched the TV on without changing the channel, then sat down on the floor in front of it and began to cry.

As the picture cleared, I saw a woman pointing her finger straight at me and saying, "I believe in miracles." I said aloud, simply, "So do I." I had never heard of Kathryn Kuhlman before, but her broadcast impressed me more than I can say. From that moment on, I had hope. I took the family Bible to bed that night and reread every miracle our Lord had ever performed.

A few days later Chris was unplugged from most of his equipment and was eating solid food. Surely, we would not have seen that gleam in his eye if he knew the prognosis of his case. Dr. Crandall introduced us to the doctor who was head of U.C.L.A.'s Radiation Therapy, Dr. Edward Langdon, one of the warmest people I have ever met. He came up to Chris' floor and told us that they had decided to start Chris on cobalt treatments as soon as possible. They hoped to shrink the tumor and prolong Chris' days on this earth. They made it perfectly clear that the treatments would not be curative, but they were quite excited about recent results of their newest methods. I asked them how many treatments they predicted Chris would need, and they estimated he would have one every single day for about six weeks. This meant, of course, making the long trip on the freeway every day right into the middle of June. This was such a shock to us and we wondered how we'd ever tell Chris. Even before this news, we had been having a terrible problem keeping our secret. Every day a team of doctors and students visited Chris' room and talked rather freely about the case. Now, when the idea of cobalt treatments was introduced, another problem presented itself. I was sure he'd know everything as soon as he got one look at that machine. So, we decided to go one step further and try to brazen it through. The doctor who was head of the Radiation Therapy Department was one of the few who sided with us and wanted to spare

Chris the awful truth. He took me down to the Radiation Therapy Department and I scanned the walls and doors for any sign which read "Cancer" or "Cobalt." There were none. Even the very machine under which the boy would lie bore no telltale markings. Only a small directional arrow pointing to the "Radiation Therapy Department" gave me a problem. I decided, with Bill, to try and turn it into something positive . . . and the good doctor, along with all the others in that department agreed to help. We told Chris that someday, in a week or so, he would have a few radiation (or heat) treatments —a normal procedure in the case of cranial operations. It was just a precaution, we said, to speed up the internal healing process. He seemed to believe us.

In the next few days, he began getting up on the side of the bed and taking a few steps around the room. Then, one wonderful day, he took his first walk down the hall. In the Neuropsychiatric Wing there are railings down both sides of the hall, but in keeping with his wonderful determined spirit Chris would have no part of them. He insisted on walking, unassisted, right down the middle of the hall. A nurse walked beside him, but without touching him. As I stood in the door of his room, watching his faltering steps, his bony legs under the blue bathrobe, amazed that he could even balance that giant turban on his frail shoulders, I said to myself, "He's going to make it! If anyone can do it, Chris can!"

45

We were pleasantly surprised one morning to discover that the bandages had been removed. He was sitting up in bed, with a knitted hospital cap covering the scars, and he was very cheerful. Normal color had returned to his face, and he really looked like our little "Creep" again. "Wow," we all said, "you look great!" His face clouded for a moment. "They're going to take the stitches out tomorrow," he said. "There are fifty-six of them!" It was an accusation! "You told me it was just a little operation!" "Well, Honey," I stumbled, "it turned out to be a pretty large tumor. You're a very lucky boy." He was a boy who loved science and knew quite a bit about the human anatomy. I expected a barrage of questions, but instead, he simply said, "Thank God for Dr. Crandall. He saved my life." Never from that day did he neglect to say the same small prayer at bedtime.

A few days later, after a short delay, the stitches were removed. I was shocked to see the huge horseshoe scar running from the base of one ear over the back of his head to the base of the other ear. There were three or four nasty holes, or clamp marks, and on the right-hand side of his head a rather large V-shaped scar where the shunt had been attached. This tube was clearly visible just under the skin, running down behind his right ear and terminating at the point marked by a three-inch scar on his throat. Of course, he couldn't see the shunt since it was behind his ear—but I was sure he would feel it eventually.

We were a little disappointed not to have been there to bolster his morale, but the stitches were removed by the time we arrived at 9:30 A.M. (I must mention here, with gratitude to the personnel on his hall, that they allowed us to come in as early as we could and stay as late as Chris could tolerate. He was the only child in that wing, and I'm sure both the nature of his case and his cheerful determination endeared him to everyone.) Chris was quite chipper over losing his stitches. I'm sure he felt a little more removed from the hospital, and a little nearer to home.

He now insisted on walking the length of the hall and around the corner to his original room to visit his friend. There was another chess game that day, and for the first time we noticed that his laugh had turned inside-out. Instead of pushing out air (ha-ha), he would suck it in, in funny big gulps that seemed to reach right to the "gut." He never lost this most engaging laugh, nor could we ever hear it without joining in. We used to kid him that everything came out just fine, except that the surgeon made a mistake and turned his laugh inside-out.

One day, after we had been sitting in his room for hours, reading, joking and watching TV, Bill and the boys went down to the cafeteria for a bite to eat. Out of a dead silence, Chris said to me, "Mom, what does terminal mean?" My insides turned to ice. Someone had let the word drop. My answer was stupid and hardly believable. I looked him straight

47

in the eye and said, "Terminal? Gee, I don't know. What have you been reading?" "It's not anything I was reading," he replied. "I just heard it—and they were talking about me." "Well," I returned, "the only terminal I can think of is a bus terminal. I'm sure they weren't talking about you." He insisted they were. He was getting angry. "Well," I faltered, "to terminate means to end something. I guess that means the end of your tumor and the end of your troubles, but just to reassure you, I'll ask your doctors." We never mentioned the word again. But I found as the months went on that it seemed to turn up on every other TV show and in every morning newspaper, and we had to screen everything that came into his view in the hospital and later at home.

After he had been in his private room for about a week, Chris began his cobalt treatments. Chris described the big machine he had to lie under, but said the treatment took only a minute and that there was nothing to it. He was making steady improvement. Three digested meals a day and a lot of rest made him look better than he had in years. It was impossible for me to believe that such a horrible thing was growing inside his little head.

The doctors decided at that time that company would be good for him, so they moved him to a four-bed suite down the hall. It was quite a move since Chris had again accumulated a tremendous assortment of gifts, cards, and posters. Instead of complaining about the clutter, or asking us to take some of it home, the wonderful group of nurses decorated his corner without omitting a single thing. We would have kept Chris in the private room, but the doctors explained that it was needed for more recent surgeries. But Chris was delighted! Another move toward recovery! Unfortunately, it wasn't. The third night in the new room, during dinner, he began to talk thick-tongued, and to have difficulty swallowing. Within minutes the doctors were at his bedside. They explained that it was a rather rare reaction to the cobalt—a swelling of the mouth and throat—and they made rapid plans to insert a tube to aid him in breathing. Poor Chris became panicky as they ran for the tray of instruments. I promised Chris that I'd try to stay and hold his hand, but I never got a chance to ask. I was propelled out into the hall and the door closed behind me. Three words came clearly through that closed door, the only words of discouragement I ever heard Chris utter: "God, why me?" I sat down on the floor in the hall and sobbed. I'd have given anything to have Bill there. An eternity or two later, the "icy" doctor (the only one with whom I never got along) came out and told me with an angry edge on his voice that Chris wouldn't cooperate and they couldn't get the tube down his throat. I felt like applauding. The swelling began to subside almost at once, and Chris finished his dinner in fine style.

Grandpa and Grandma, who had extended their stay by several weeks to see us through the worst of it, went home to Rochester. Chris was terribly saddened at their leaving. By now, however, the doctors were beginning to talk about a date for Chris' release. He was now out of bed for long periods each day, and on several occasions was permitted to go for a long wheel-chair ride down to the main lobby. After some six weeks in the confinement of four walls, it was a real treat for him to browse through the gift shop, or wheel through the cafeteria, choosing anything he wanted to eat. During the very last week of his stay we never went to lunch or dinner without him. Though the bulk of his meals were eaten in his room, they encouraged him to eat all the between-meal snacks he wanted and his wheelchair was always at the end of our table. Chris looked great to us, but the shaved head under the hospital cap revealed that he was a brain-surgery patient, and the sight of him provoked looks of both horror and pathos on the faces of strangers.

We never understood why Chris himself was not more visibly alarmed at the sight of his bald head and the purple cobalt markings up the back of his neck. Later, when he was home, he insisted on accompanying me to the stores, library, and often suggested we go out to dinner as a family. I like to think he was just so glad to be alive that appearance didn't matter much any more. But it could be that he knew the whole truth all the time, and just wanted to drink in as much of this life as possible before he had to come to grips with the next.

50

The going home date was postponed several times. Chris was getting itchy. Twice when we were leaving him at night he said to me, "Mom, I'm scared." I said, "What can you possibly be scared about now? You've been through all the most frightening things, Hon. Now it's just a matter of another day or two of rest." God! How I hated to leave him those last few nights. Fortunately a pleasant U.C.L.A. medical student stayed with Chris, and the two would listen to a ball game on the radio until Chris fell asleep. One night I packed Chris' suitcase and brought it up to him, just to give him a boost. When the doctors saw the suitcase, they made a joke of it. "Hey, Chris, why didn't you tell us you wanted to go home? Suppose we make it tomorrow!" I've never seen a face light up as his did.

The next morning was almost a fiasco! Bill had an important meeting and just couldn't take time off. His company had been most generous as it was those past several weeks. Mark was studying hard for final exams before he was to graduate from high school. That left me with one sixteen-year-old driver (though Kev was very capable), and an old broken-down Ford Galaxie. The thought of postponing the homecoming for one day crossed our minds, but it didn't linger long. We couldn't disappoint Chris. So we decided that we'd make a bed in the back seat. I'd drive up and Kev would drive home, while I attended to Chris. Not discounting all of the light-hearted good times we'd had in the past, this was one of the happiest days of our lives.

A look of great relief crossed Chris' face when we entered his room. He was sitting up on the side of his bed, fully dressed, and finishing his breakfast. While the doctor signed his release, Kev and I made several trips down to the car with all of Chris' gear. Many of the doctors and nurses turned out for the send-off, some of them fighting back tears. Chris asked one of the nurses for a scissors. With some help, he snipped off his plastic hospital I.D. bracelet. "Don't you want to keep it for a souvenir?" one of the girls asked. "No, thank you," he replied with a sheepish grin, "I want you to have it."

He shoved aside our bed in the back seat and sat up all the way home, relishing the sight of every car, every bit of scenery. At last we pulled into our street, a short cul-de-sac which bends into a corkscrew in such a way that our house can't be seen until you are upon it. Unknown to all of us, Dale, the boy across the street and Chris' best friend, had fashioned a red carpet all the way up our driveway. A huge sign above it read; "WELCOME HOME, CHRIS." At first sight of it, Chris broke down and cried like a baby.

4

The Burden of Hope

We were pretty sure that Chris was not crying from a broken heart but from plain relief. What an ordeal for a fourteen-year-old! He had endured great apprehension, terror, and pain. But for the moment, it didn't matter. As in any crisis, one chooses to believe what one wants. We had not robbed him of this privilege. He was home!

I thought he'd want to tour the whole house to see how it was changed in his absence, but the trip home must have taken more out of him than we realized, for he plunked himself down in a big living-room chair and seemed quite content to stay put. A few of the neighborhood kids, some on half-day school sessions because of exams, were into the house immediately! Dale, of course—the "red carpet" boy—three boys from the next street, and the little girls across from us. One of the girls (Jeannie) baked Chris some homemade oatmeal cookies and he ate not less than fifteen of them, with several glasses of milk. His happiness radiated around the room while the kids made all kinds of plans for his first dip in their pools, a little ping-pong tournament in the garage, and later on, a triumphant visit to Disneyland.

Chris loved his own room with all his private mementos. However, unknown to him, we had made plans to put him in Mark's room, downstairs. He would have his own bath, and a low-hanging window that looks out on the front yard. The room opened directly onto a large carpeted rumpus room, with color television, and a level exit to the back yard patio. While resting in bed, Chris could watch the ballplayers in the street. He could get up and entertain his guests in the rumpus room, and eat his dinner in front of the TV. Upstairs in his old room he would have been much more confined. The windows are high and the stairs are steep.

After an hour and a half of his homecoming party, Chris began to tire. I helped him downstairs, and he seemed delighted with his new room. The bed had been prepared, crisp and white. An early afternoon breeze whispered through the window, and with great nonchalance, he agreed to take a short rest—if I insisted. I cannot express my feelings of peace at seeing him safely in bed, where no doctors ruled, where no needles threatened, where only love abided. He had a light lunch and settled back. But it soon became apparent that he

54

was far too excited to sleep. He wanted to talk about anything and everything. He was concerned mainly about school. The doctors had discouraged us from bringing his books to the hospital, even though Chris had asked for them several times. Only four weeks remained in the school year. Chris was to graduate from Ridgecrest Intermediate School and enter Rolling Hills High School, where his brothers were already enrolled. Chris had an excellent record at Ridgecrest, and although he had been out of school since the first part of April, his teachers had already assured us that he would graduate. But still it bothered him greatly. He was independent and didn't want any charity. He wanted to take his final exams.

I slept on a cot just outside his room. The first night home was long and wakeful. Chris was disturbed by the prospect of starting the next morning—and each subsequent morning—with a trip to the hospital for his cobalt treatments.

As I have mentioned, the U.C.L.A. Radiation Therapy Department is in the basement of the hospital, at the far end of a gloomy concrete corridor. Just at the corner, where two corridors meet, a long row of chairs line the wall. Here, sitting not so patiently for their various types of therapy, are the people, a disheartening sampling of humanity—some old and sick, some young and beautiful, some who have not yet been to kindergarten. They were the victims of one of nature's cruelest accidents; Chris was one of them. Before

55

every treatment we reported to the lab where a blood sample was taken. Many times, after an hour on the freeway, a wait in the lab, and another wait for the results of the test, they'd find Chris' blood count to be too low for a treatment. After many weeks of this, we obtained permission to have the blood tests done early in the morning at a lab near our home. The lab would phone the results of the test to the cobalt room, and we would then be called at home and told whether to bring Chris in for treatment.

The freeway traffic was heavy in the early morning, but not so bad at noon. The cobalt room traffic was just the opposite. There were no appointments; it was first come, first served, with a lot of hospital in-patients being fitted in between. We played "Beat the cobalt crowd," and played it in every way possible. When we arrived at U.C.L.A. each day, I had to make a dash for the lobby to get a wheel chair. Then, back to the car to pick up Chris. Someone ought to do something about the parking situation at that place. There is a parking lot out front where you pay your dollar and stay all day, but the Radiation Therapy Department is roughly one mile from that lot. The parking meters in back allow you to deposit only one quarter at a time for twenty-five minutes. The Radiation Therapy Department is a ten-minute walk from there, and we rarely had less than a two-hour wait, no matter how we cut it.

There was much commotion in the hallway.

Many of the older patients wanted to talk "cancer" all the time. Doctors were constantly conferring with relatives of patients, openly, in the hall. I was trying to spare Chris all of this, but it was difficult. I never wanted to leave him waiting there alone while I ran all the way back to put another quarter in the meter; I paid a good number of parking fines. After a time, we discovered a waiting room way down the hall. It was usually empty. I left Chris there with some good books from home and a little candy or a soft drink while I waited in line until his turn came up. This went on every day into June and much beyond.

Three days before graduation, we learned that Daddy's sister, Grace, and Grandma McIvers were coming out from New York for the event. Before we knew of their coming, we had decided that the best graduation gift outside of a few trinkets, would be a long weekend at our beloved Lake Arrowhead. The people at the hospital concurred and gave Chris a few days' rest from his treatments. So we consulted a realtor, and rented a nice four-bedroom house. With company arriving, we decided to throw in a few sleeping bags and take the whole crowd along. On their arrival, Grace and Grandma were openly shocked at Chris' appearance, and didn't sleep a wink that night, though they claimed to feel reassured with the way we were handling the situation. The preparations for graduation and for the trip went along as lightheartedly as if we had no problems at all.

We planned quite a graduation party. It was a double graduation, with Mark graduating from Rolling Hills High School, and Chris from Ridgecrest Intermediate School. We were allowed just three tickets to the graduation exercises, and since Chris was too weak to attend his own ceremony, we decided that Dad, Grandma, and myself would be present at Mark's. Aunt Grace (who is a nurse), Kevin, and Chris were elected to stay at home and set up the buffet table for later festivities.

The graduation exercises were held in a lovely outdoor amphitheater, and Mark, looking magnificent in his blue cap and gown, played in the high school orchestra for a good part of the ceremony. We were so proud and happy, doubly proud knowing that Kev would be graduating the following year from the same stage, but saddened to think that our darling Chris would almost surely never make it to the platform.

Silly, I guess, the way your mind wanders, but I thought as I sat there that I had always wanted six or seven children. I could only have three—and all of those by Caesarean section. Why, then, was God taking one away from us? Had we not loved him enough? But what of the battered children? What of all the starving children? Someday, in God's good time, we will know the answer.

When the ceremony was over the neighbors all turned out for a buffet supper, climaxed by a big graduation cake in blue and gold, with the words, "CONGRATULATIONS, MARK AND CHRIS" scrawled across the top. The two boys shared the spotlight as they opened gifts and accepted best wishes, but the real center of attention was Chris, diploma tacked up on the very top of the lid of our grand piano. We all knew it was the last one he would ever receive.

The next morning, bright and early, we took off for the San Bernardino Mountains in two cars. It was one of the hottest days I could remember, and in our old cars, sans air conditioning, we sweltered all the way up. In the back seat, poor Grandma was really suffering, and I kept assuring her that just as soon as we started up the mountain, it would be cooler. Lake Arrowhead is approximately 5,000 feet up, and when we finally arrived at the top, the temperature had not varied one degree.

The house we had rented was even more beautiful than described, but there were a few drawbacks. It was miles from the lake; the deck was on the hot, sunny side of the house, therefore unusable. They were cutting through a new road right next to the house, and every morning the huge watering trucks and earth movers put an abrupt end to our night's sleep. The weekend was a disappointment, though not a total loss, since we did manage to drive around the lake, visit the candy shop, and make grandiose plans for another summer vacation.

Chris' condition declined in the following weeks. The cobalt was troubling him and his eating fell off abruptly. His vomiting returned. About the second week home, however, his hair began to grow in. Since it was quite black, it didn't take much growth to camouflage the scars and give the appearance of a crew cut. We had been trying to take things one step at a time, and now, in the midst of his excitement over his new hair, I had to tell him that the cobalt would shortly cause it to fall out again. He took the news without flinching. He only wanted to know how long he'd have to wait before it came back again. When the hair got to be about an inch long, the process began, and there was quite a problem keeping the little black "prickles" out of his bed and out from around the the neck of his T-shirts. During the time of the treatments, he was not supposed to get any sun on his head, so we bought him several caps and hats, but he wore a little black knitted cap (Bronson style), most of the time.

By the end of June, 1970, we had fallen into a regular pattern. He'd start out each morning with breakfast in bed. I kidded him about everything and he gave it right back. Mornings were the worst time for eating, and I used to tell him that if I didn't know better I'd think he was pregnant. He kept down just about everything that he ate in bed. Dressing was slow and I had to split many of his shirts to get them over his sensitive head.

Next, it was a quick trip down to the lab. By now, the poor dear was like a pin-cushion, and they were having difficulty finding a place to insert the needle. But he never peeped about it and always left the nurse laughing. I remember one morning in particular, when we were at the lab. A young girl whom Chris had known in better days came into the office to have some blood drawn. Of course, she knew nothing of Chris' ordeal. She was very nervous, and Chris laughed and reassured her, "Don't worry, I did it once; there's nothing to it."

We then came home and had a pleasant interlude, lingering over a second breakfast, and hashing over the morning paper. When a positive call came from the hospital, we started out. I could never say enough about the car trouble we had in those days. Our budget was stretched beyond all imagination. I was always making calls asking for more time, or paying ridiculously small amounts just to keep out of the credit bureau. And still the cars blew tires, boiled over, needed brakes. One awful morning, I took the car over to the local ARCO station before braving the freeway. I had all but kept that station in business for the past year. When the mechanic told me that the car couldn't be driven on the freeway without an additional $68.00 in work, I broke down and cried. He never knew the extent of our problems; I guess he thought I was crazy.

I often drove onto the freeway knowing full well that the car was unsafe. Bill used to worry about it, too, but I told him the good Lord had to be on our side. How could I have a blowout while taking a dying child for a cobalt treatment? I guess God was there, all right. He didn't pay the bills, but we always made it home safely.

After the treatments, it was a good day if we got home by two o'clock. Chris loved to eat out, though it gave me the "woolies" wondering whether or not he could keep the food down. Of course, I never mentioned this to him, but went out of my way choosing a table or booth near the men's room. One rare day, he ate a whole shrimp dinner and a strawberry shortcake at Howard Johnson's. I was so thrilled that I could have kissed the cook! The treatment, combined with the long, hot ride always knocked him out, and he lay down for most of the afternoon. He always wanted to just flop on the bed, clothes and all. The days were so hot that I wanted him to take his clothes off and slip in between cool sheets. We laughingly referred to that as a bona-fide nap. As to who won—it was about fifty-fifty.

Bill's coming home was always a happy relief for Chris, who pumped his dad full of questions about the things he had done all day. At this particular time, Dad's office was below ground level, and apparently a small stray fox had wandered by the window one day. There were great jokes about Dad spending his days feeding the fox. No doubt, this basement office really bothered Chris, who always took the greatest interest in all of us. He worried about Kev's and Mark's grades, about my smoking, and about Dad's office. Dad used to kid and tell him that they hadn't given him a new office as yet, but that he had been presented with an "executive wastebasket." This always brought about that inside-out chuckle which so endeared Chrisie to all of us.

After quite a few minutes of happy chatter, we'd always give one of the other boys the "high-sign" to take over, and Dad and I would meet in the garage. After the usual questions—"How did it go today?" "What did they have to say at the hospital?"—we'd invariably throw our arms around each other and cry our eyes out. We would keep saying over and over, "I don't believe it; It can't be happening to us."

By this time, I had become quite interested in Kathryn Kuhlman, and in those desperate moments, I tried to impart to Bill some of the hope I had found through her telecasts, but he was so skeptical he didn't even want to hear about it. On some Sunday mornings I'd pry Bill loose from his newspaper to hear one of her telecasts, a case that closely paralleled ours. Sometimes he listened, but he never believed it.

Those nightly crying sessions were actually a relief, having gone around all day with a lump in my throat, fighting back tears. But soon we would remind ourselves that Chris would notice if we were all cried up, and we would return to the kitchen and make a drink. Bill would change his clothes and have his drink in Chris' room while they watched the nightly news. I sipped my drink while putting the finishing touches on dinner, this ritual having become a laugh. Chris ate lobster in the rumpus room; we ate pea soup in the kitchen. But he was seldom aware of this.

After dinner things livened up a little. Someone usually got out the chessboard, while another made popcorn or fudge. During those precious moments we made it a point to bring the outside world in to Chris, with each of us conjuring up any funny little anecdote that had happened during the day, sometimes embellishing it until it became unrecognizable; anything to lighten his heart.

The nights were still long and wakeful. For some reason, Chris craved hot chocolate, a beverage he had never particularly liked in the past. He drank at least six cups at intervals during the night, each accompanied by long conversation. He was happy, and had great plans for the future. He mentioned several times his desire to attend Cornell University at Ithaca, New York, a spot he had visited with his dad many times in the happy past. In between hot chocolates, I would lie on my little cot, alternately praying and sobbing, sometimes so loudly that I had to hide my head under the pillow. My mind was bursting with fatigue and worry, and I used to come up with dumb little jingles that I couldn't seem to stifle:

> "Someone is dying in our house
> Someone who's too young to go.
> Christopher's going to leave us,
> And all of us love him so."

If I were lucky, sleep would overtake me for an hour or two. Then it was back to the daytime routine: getting the boys off to school, Dad off to work, Chris to the lab and the hospital.

One morning when we came around the corner to the cobalt room, everyone broke into simultaneous applause. Chris was without his wheel chair, having walked the whole long route from the parking lot. He had leaned on me all the way to the corner of the hall, then, shaking me off, with head in the air, shoulders back, he marched straight down the middle of that hall, exuding such confidence that one might have expected him to break into a run.

In August of 1970, a new member joined our family, and if ever there was a small miracle she was one of them. Chris had always wanted a sheltie dog—a miniature collie. This particular day, he took a notion to scan the want ads and find one. There were three advertisements offering sheltie puppies. We called the first two, and found that the going price was somewhere between $125 and $150. It hurt me to say no, but we gave him the choice of saving up for one, or getting a little mongrel from the Humane Society. But Chris was determined to call the last ad, even though I warned him against being disappointed. On the last call, he talked to a woman, who, bless her heart, will never know what she did for us. It seems she had some twenty shelties, and was, I believe, dissolving her kennels. She offered Chris the most beautiful little female, free, on a co-ownership basis, i.e., that if we ever wanted to breed the dog, she would choose the stud and have first pick of the litter. Chris was in seventh heaven.

The next day, we went out to pick up the pup. Chris received all the pedigree papers, and a whole handful of ribbons and first-place trophies the dog had won. On the way home, Chris rode in the back with "Vicki," and she was strictly his dog from that moment on. She played when he felt up to it, she lay at his feet while he did homework, and if he had a bad day or two, she never left her spot at the foot of his bed.

By the end of the summer, Chris was getting around pretty well. We were amazed at his coordination in playing ping-pong. In August, we obtained another leave from the treatments (which still took up our every day), and returned to our beloved Lake Arrowhead, this time renting a house directly above the lake. Don't ask me where we got the money. We only knew Chris' time was short, and we had to go. He wasn't supposed to be out in the sun, but we amused him during the day with mild hiking, feeding the wildlife he loved so well, and just watching water-skiers from the lovely shaded deck. He was allowed to go in the water but not get his head wet, so we saved our swimming time until dusk and invented many water games in which we all participated. The neatest participant was "Vicki," who just loved the water, and accompanied Chris everywhere. The older boys had jobs that summer, but came for a day or two whenever they were free, often bringing a few friends.

We also made our annual trip to the village,

where each little shop was charmingly patterned after a Swiss chalet. In the past, it had always been an adventure to visit the penny arcade, play a round on the miniature golf course, take a boat ride, and sample some of the delicacies at the homemade candy shop. The kids' favorites had always been caramel apples and rock candy. The caramel apples were for eating, then and there. The rock candy was for later. When this vacation was over and we arrived home, Chris, as always, tucked a little bag of rock candy into his desk drawer.

It was the middle of October 1970 before we heard the good news that his treatments were nearing an end. They had given him the maximum dosage he could tolerate. One hundred and three treatments in all! Of course, it was going to be a tremendous relief not to have to make that grueling trip to U.C.L.A. every day, but when the final day arrived, I had mixed emotions. As he lay under that huge machine, and I watched him, as always, on the little monitor outside the room, I had a terrible sinking feeling that they had done all they could for him, and from now on the whole responsibility lay squarely on our shoulders. There were, again, farewells to be said, but believe me, they were brief. Chris couldn't wait to get out of there.

He was ecstatic all the way home. We bought a slurpy; he was free!

5

Oh, God! Let Him Live a Little!

Dr. Crandall examined Chris a month after his release from the cobalt treatments. While he put Chris through the usual neurological tests, his expression revealed that he was happy with Chris' progress. At the end of the examination, he asked Chris, "How are you feeling?" "Foin," was the answer. "Any problems?" asked the doctor. "None," Chris volleyed. "Any questions?" "Yes," replied Chris, hiding a grin, "can I ride my skate-board?" The doctor smiled broadly. "No," he said. The next visit in November he said, "Yes."

While the nurse weighed and measured Chris, the doctor took me aside and told me that from all indications, "that thing" had shrunk to "nothing." With a little luck, he would now give Chris five to eight years. Then he added, "Maybe fifteen." I apologized profusely for what I had said on that awful day in the conference room. I was so ashamed, and so glad he hadn't "slipped." Now, for the first time in over three years, my hopes were almost substantiated. I thought of Kathryn Kuhlman, I thought of God, I even thought of Vicki. The miracles were beginning to happen!

Early that fall, I opened the morning paper and was delighted to see that Kathryn Kuhlman was coming to the Shrine Auditorium in Los Angeles. I had no idea at that time that she came regularly. Neither did I have any conception of the magnitude of her following. The ad in the paper said the doors would open at 1:00 P.M. the following Sunday. On the many telecasts, which I faithfully watched, the people giving accounts of miracles always mentioned that they were in the audience when they were healed. I knew the program came from Pittsburgh, and I had many times thought of going there. To discover that she was actually going to come to within a half hour of our house thrilled me. Bill wasn't at all in favor of my going, but he was supportive, and I was determined. When I arrived at the Shrine Auditorium next Sunday, I was astounded to find literally thousands of people jamming the doors, the street, and the adjacent parking lots. Parking took forever, and by the time I ran a good distance back to the area of the front doors, I was told that the doors had already opened, and the crowd that surrounded me was the overflow. I was sorely disappointed, but I knelt down on the pavement with hundreds of others and listened to her message over the loud speakers. I prayed so hard, and cried so much, that I was convinced of finding Chris cured when I returned home at 4:00 P.M. The next time Miss Kuhlman appeared at Shrine Auditorium I was at the doors before ten in the morning. I can never tell you how impressed I was with that beautiful service. I saw miracles! Dozens of them! I will be convinced of this until the day I die. Over the next two years, I never missed a service. I must have attended some twenty times, taking each one of the family with me, in turn, including Chris.

The first one to accompany me to the Kathryn Kuhlman service was Kevin. We packed a lunch and arrived at the doors somewhere around 10:00 A.M. If you arrived any later, you are almost certain not to get inside. While waiting, many people gathered into little groups and sang hymns or read aloud from the Bible. When the doors finally opened we were stampeded into the hall, like cattle to the slaughterhouse. We found a seat in the second balcony, and waited another half hour until, with a musical crescendo, Miss Kuhlman appeared on stage. I was hoping Kev would be as impressed as I had been in the past, but a couple of things turned him off. There is a great deal of pageantry and theatrical gyrations involved in the show. This, compared with the quiet simplicity of Christ's life, seemed to Kev to be out of place at a religious service. We sat directly across the aisle from a very sickly looking old man. When the miracles began to happen, Miss Kuhlman was calling for people with back trouble to stand up and take their healing. The old man dragged himself to his feet. He was obviously in great pain. After a minute passed, he eased himself back into his seat, but Miss Kuhlman was still curing back problems, and she continued to call for people with any back ailment to get to their feet. At least five times this poor soul across the aisle pulled himself to his feet, and painfully sat down again, tears streaming down his face. Kev was so touched by this that he never could forgive Miss Kuhlman for giving people false hope and then sending them home dejected. He was so hurt over this old man that I'm sure he missed seeing the real miracles that happened that day.

The next one to visit the Kathryn Kuhlman service with me was Mark. He had been quite turned off by Kevin's reaction but was curious enough to see what this pageantry was all about. We had also told him that when Miss Kuhlman lays hands on a person they fall to the floor in what seems to be a dead faint. Mark just couldn't believe this; he had to see it for himself. So Mark and I made the trip. Mark's reaction was much the same as Kevin's: too much "window dressing." Mark had always been quite a student of the Bible and he pointed out to me all the way home that Jesus was a simple man, and that his apostles were chosen for their simplicity of life style. He was not as closed-minded as Kev, however. He was impressed with the caliber of the guests on stage: doctors, ministers, priests. He thought the miracles possible.

There was a lot of comparing of notes when we got home. Both boys concurred that if God wanted to heal Chris, He would do it right there at home, without benefit of the grand pianos, Miss Kuhlman's flowing white dress, and all the "Praise the Lords." They made it clear they would not accompany me there again.

Bill thought I was completely given over to emotionalism, dreams, false hopes. Of course, I continued to go to our church every day, and I distinctly remember Bill shouting at me once, "Why are you such a hypocrite?" Bill, a quietly religious man, felt that we had found a path to God through our own church, and needed no outside influences to call God's attention to our needs. Bill was very upset with me over the whole Kuhlman experience and he didn't like involving the boys.

I must try to tell you some of my reasons for going against my husband's wishes. I was sure that many people were healed at these services. But, as in the case of the old man, not all were healed. Miss Kuhlman will be the first to tell you that she does not know the reason for this, and that she is often troubled by it. I had it in the back of my head, however, that perhaps I didn't know how to pray in the way God wanted. Perhaps I wasn't worthy of his attention. I had hopes that maybe God would listen to Kevin or Mark. You must try to realize the degree of our desperation at this point. Time was running out, and I have to admit that I had never in my life seen a miracle in our Catholic Church, or in any other.

But I believe to this day that the miracles I saw performed by Miss Kuhlman were real beyond a doubt, and that she is, in a special way, in touch with the Holy Spirit. In every case that I have been privileged to witness the miracles were fully documented. Miss Kuhlman always encouraged the miraculously cured to go back to their doctors and have a complete physical, and I have heard the testimonies of countless doctors who could not believe the most recent set of X-rays on terminal patients. Ever-present on her stage were great men of both the medical and religious professions. I have thrilled to see the sick and crippled from the City of Hope, Stanford Medical Center, U.C.L.A., from all over the country and the world, who were brought in on stretchers or in wheelchairs get up and leap through the aisles, thankful and incredulous. For me, it was no longer a case of "believing" in her miracles. I knew what I had seen.

In November, 1970, another wonderful thing happened. Chris started with a home teacher. This one was a jewel, one of the nicest, most cheerful, most patient people I've ever encountered, Mrs. Beverly Peterson. With Chris' stomach giving him problems, and with all of his friends in school all day, time often dragged for him, but when this sterling lady came in the front door, she brought the sunshine with her. She never failed to have a little joke, a cheerful word, or a cute anecdote about her own wonderful family. She was truly the bright spot of our day. Because Chris had missed too much school (from March to November, 1970), he was not recommended for Algebra I, but for Algebra Prep. After a couple of months of careful coaching, this wonderful woman gave him the Algebra Prep test and moved him to Algebra I, which he passed the following June with flying colors.

But if there were great gains, there were also losses. Dale, the red carpet boy, was Chris' best friend. Every afternoon, he used to come over after school and kid Chris out of his long nap, sit for a good half hour while Chris drank his "loaded" milkshake, and then either practice golf on the back lawn, or get a late date at Los Verdes Golf Course. With the doctor's permission, Chris had started golf lessons at the Rolling Hills Golf Club. Dale had been playing regularly and Chris thought he needed a few lessons to catch up with him. Though he was a "lefty," playing with an old set of right-handed clubs, he did remarkably well. I have the pro's word for that. He got quite interested in Chris and gave him three or four free lessons.

Dale was one of the very few people who knew Chris' whole story, but he never gave the slightest indication that he considered Chris anything but robust and healthy.

It was quite a blow when we learned that Dale was moving to Louisiana. On the day of the move, after all the goodbyes had been said, Chris was out in the side yard in his little black cap, his frail frame hunched over a golf club. If ever I saw a hint of dejection on his face, or a slight slump to his shoulders, it was at that moment when the moving truck made a wide arc in the cul-de-sac, and pulled out of sight.

But the glorious season of Christmas was upon us again. We wanted to do something extra special for Chris. With Dale gone, his interest in golf had waned. Most of Chris' school friends no longer came around, except for the nice girls across the street. Chris told us he wanted something that he could do by himself, namely, movie equipment. I had been trying to persuade him to get a ten-speed bike because I hoped the exercise would build him up. But he persisted. The price of projectors being what they were, we found a good Bell & Howell at a pawn shop. We bought a little new camera and got the screen with Blue Chip Stamps.

But, when we discovered that two of Chris' friends were getting ten-speeds, we bought a ten-speed for Chris and hid it in a neighbor's garage. The thought that he might not be around next year kept haunting me.

It was a great Christmas! We did all the old things again: baked two hundred Christmas cookies, watched Dickens' "Christmas Carol," went to Midnight Mass at the same church, played a lot of music, opened numerous presents and ate pounds of turkey. We also took a lot of movies with Chris' new camera, though I've not been able to look at them to this day.

One sweet thing I remember so well about that Christmas was that Chris's voice was changing. That year Chris got a kick out of singing, "Hark, the Herald Angels Sing." When he got to the next line, "Glory . . . ," his voice would crack miserably, and we'd shout from all corners of the house, "For God's sake, don't sing, you'll ruin the whole holiday!" Then that inside-out chuckle would fill the house. It was a sound lovelier than the most melodic carol.

My heart broke at the sweet sound—a man, but still a boy. Never a girl friend, never a driver's license, never a chance to master Cornell, or match his wits with life. Again, my jingles haunted me:

> All through the long gray winter . . .
> All through the lush green spring,
> All through the silent summer . . .
> I'll never hear him sing.

There had been quite a few petty thefts in our neighborhood that winter, so Bill insisted Chris keep his new bike in the rumpus room at least until after the holidays. The day after the tree came down, we moved it to the garage. The next day it was gone. We never saw it again, and we couldn't afford to replace it.

The boys went back to school, and Chris back to his home teacher. He was doing very well indeed. In other things, too; the neighbors used to cringe when he hopped on his skate-board, headed full-speed down our steep driveway, and rounded the corner, missing the sharp corner of our mailbox by an inch. But we had to let him do it! We had to let him do everything he could. His little black cap was on the shelf now, and the horrible scars were again out of sight. He made Dad and me sign a paper stating that we would never, ever, make him get a haircut as long as he lived. We never did.

Of course, we wanted him to see as much and do as much as possible in whatever time he had left. We would have done so much more if we had the means. Dad took Chris on a nice business trip to San Francisco. It was the first time he had seen that city, and also his first plane ride. He was slightly sick on the jet, but Dad assured me it didn't dampen his spirits at all. They went everywhere and saw everything and when they came home, they were bubbling with conversation.

Another delightful father and son experience was a trip to San Diego, where they stayed at the old Del Coronado Hotel. The pool wasn't heated, but Chris insisted on going in anyway, and stayed until Dad had to beg him to get out. They were two of a kind, he and Dad, in many ways, though I would say that Chris was more outgoing and fun-loving. However, they both were men of few words and had a quiet rapport that we all recognized. Both had an insatiable appetite for the printed word, and even Bill will admit that Chris could talk intelligently on almost any subject.

As a matter of fact, Chris was interested in anything and everything. When Chris was four or five, we had many an opportunity to take small trips with Dad when he travelled the East Coast on business. Chris would stand up in the back seat of the car, his arms wrapped around Bill's neck, and ask questions from the time we left the house until our return a few days later. One of his pet phrases was, "Tell me more, Dad. Tell me all about it." Sometimes, if Dad didn't know all about a given subject, he'd come up with a rather vague generalization, followed by a half apology that he "may not have hit the nail exactly on the head, but was at least in the ballpark." As years went by, and the boys became more knowledgeable on a number of topics than the "old man," they'd punctuate every question with, "and don't give us one of your ballpark answers." Dad usually answered their questions confidently and to the point. But whenever he prefaced an answer with "W-e-l-l, son," the whole gang would burst into a chorus of laughter before Dad had a chance to utter another word.

Chris had not zeroed in on any "specialty"; he still considered the world as his field. He loved sports and knew the games and the players inside-out. He had a real talent for working with his hands; the garage was his workshop. Anything electrical fascinated him, and many friends used to give him their old discarded stereos and radios, which he never failed to put into tip-top condition. He was an inveterate reader and had accumulated a backlog of knowledge on a surprising variety of subjects. He was as interested in Dad's new job as he was in Mark's faulty muffler.

He knew the value of a dollar, too. As a joke, Dad used to pay him for odd jobs in pennies. He never considered a penny unimportant, and many a day was spent on his bedroom floor rolling hundreds of them into wrappers for deposit in his personal account. He saved every penny he ever received, and besides his bank account he had a black box in his top drawer which, to the amazement of the other two boys, always had a couple of fives in it. There was something else in that little box, too—I.O.U.'s. Everyone borrowed from him—including me—and he used to amuse us no end because he wouldn't part with a buck without our signing a slip promising to pay 100% interest. Of course, it was all in fun, and none of us ever doubted that he would gladly have handed over his entire savings to anyone who needed it.

Somewhere along the way, I had promised him a lobster he had never received. Also, at some point in time, his favorite "Beatles" album, "Let It Be" had disappeared. We kind of think that one of the older boys loaned it to a friend, but no one could remember, and since I was no rock and roll lover, Chris laughingly accused me of "misplacing" it. One night about 11:00 P.M. when Bill and I were in bed and half asleep, he came into our room with a "document" he had drawn up. It read, "Mom owes me: one lobster, one "Let It Be" album, and $68.00."

We laughed until we shook the bed, because we knew there was going to be no sleep that night until I affixed my signature to that paper. I knew nothing about the album . . . but the rest was true, and I signed, resolving that, if it took my last breath, I'd fulfill the contract.

He was feeling better and better that spring of 1971. One morning, his inside-out chuckle lured me away from the morning dishes. He had found an article in the paper announcing that the "powers that be" in Rome had decided that St. Christopher —long-time patron saint of travelers—was not a saint after all. "Boy, Mom," he teased, "you really blew it this time!" Kevin and Mark, after all, were named for famous saints. Just a short time later, he found in a magazine, a "Brother Sebastian" cartoon. It pictured a plump little monk, presiding over a roadside stand in front of the monastery. The sign over the stand read, "Mr. Christopher medals —half price." From that day on, he laughingly referred to himself as "Mr. Christopher."

Chris had a recurring nightmare. He dreamed he was on a luxury liner. The sea was stormy and the deck slick. There was a low railing around the deck, and when Chris fell and slid to the very edge of the ship he grabbed onto that rail. He said that he was panicky and gasping for breath as the waves washed over him. Above him, however, on the same deck, were people dressed in formal attire, and waiters carrying huge trays of delicacies. There was music and great frivolity, but as much as he screamed for help, no one seemed to notice as he lost his grip and slipped off into the deep.

The summer of 1971 swung in hot and beautiful. Kevin graduated from high school in June. Reluctant to leave his little brother he registered at a local junior college for the fall semester. Mark would be entering his second year at the same college. We bade a sad, but triumphant goodbye to Chris' beloved home teacher, with the assurance that Chris would enter his sophomore year of high school in the fall. He took two summer school courses: health and driver's education. During this time, he renewed contacts with old friends and learned his way around the campus. When summer school was over, we went back to Lake Arrowhead. Chris was allowed to do everything, and we held our hearts in our mouths as we watched him swim right out into the middle of the lake, nearly out of sight.

Again the other boys had summer jobs—Kev at Marineland, and Mark at Hughes Market. But still, they managed to visit us on their days off, usually bringing along a friend or two. At one time, Kev brought his girl up for a few days, and Chris made welcoming signs prior to their arrival. In the downstairs hall the sign read:

KEV & JANICE
——————▶

On the stair landing, it also read:

KEV & JANICE
◀——————

81

In the upstairs hall leading to the bedrooms it changed to:

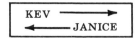

We had many laughs over this, as it was the first time we had a girl in the house overnight. Mothers don't count!

For once, coming home from a summer vacation was not a sad affair. Chris was itching to get back to school and feel "normal" for the first time in three years. Orientation Day was an important one for him. There would be the usual stations— picking up this card, dropping off that, and of course, getting pictures taken for the yearbook. I was so delighted to drop him off in front of the gym and watch as friend after friend came up and patted him on the back. Though many a kid dreaded this day, for Chris it was a big moment, his triumph after all the months of fighting! Because we felt that a full day of school would be too much for him at first, we made arrangements for Chris to take his four solid subjects in the morning so he could have lunch at home.

With bills skyrocketing, I was most fortunate in securing a part-time job at a nursery school close to home. I will always be grateful to the director of that school as I am sure no other job would have allowed me to pursue my erratic schedule.

OH, GOD! LET HIM LIVE A LITTLE!

By now, I was calling on the Deity through every possible channel. At twenty of eight in the morning, I would take Chris to school, and rush home in time to catch ten minutes of Kathryn Kuhlman on the radio at 8:00 A.M. With the Bible open to my favorite passage, I'd listen and pray for a miracle.

> "Ask, and it shall be given you; seek, and you shall find; knock, and it shall be opened to you. For everyone who asks, receives; and he who seeks, finds; and to him who knocks, it shall be opened. Or what man is there among you, who, if his son asks for a loaf, will hand him a stone; or if he asks for a fish, will hand him a serpent? Therefore, if you, evil as you are, know how to give good gifts to your children, how much more will your Father in heaven give good things to those who ask Him."
> —Mt. 7:7-11

Next was a dash over to the Catholic Church, where I was always late for the eight o'clock Mass, but in time to receive Communion. I'm sure the good Fathers wondered why I never could make it on time. From there, I went directly to nursery school until twelve o'clock, when it was time to pick Chris up at school.

I met Chris in front of the gym, where he would always linger awhile, wind up a conversation with a friend. Many times, he'd have a Coke or an ice cream he'd purchased at the snack bar. There was no doubt that he was enjoying this back-to-school experience. The fact that he was the only "crew-cut" in the midst of the "long-hairs," didn't seem to matter to anyone. All of the kids were most supportive and helpful in every way. If there was one cloud on this bright horizon, it was the fact that Chris was put into the modified physical education program, unaffectionately referred to as "Retard P. E." He was able to participate in everything except contact football, and for this reason the doctor wouldn't O.K. the regular class. But the "Retard" class played basketball, ping-pong, and went swimming.

In the afternoon, Chris usually rested for a couple of hours and then tackled his homework. During this period, I'd try to make some inroads on the housework. I recall one afternoon when I was ironing. I had just pressed a new sweatshirt of Chris' and while I was folding it and feeling its warmth, suddenly there came over me the keen contrast between it and the coldness of the grave. I buried my face in the shirt and bawled. "God," I prayed, "You wouldn't. You just couldn't, could you?" I really thought He said, "No, don't worry," and I went back to my task.

About that time, a new craze hit the neighborhood—fish! The kids were again congregating around Chris in the late afternoons, and all the talk involved tanks, filters, and tropicals. We were delighted to find a tank, complete with a lot of equipment. We started out with guppies. Boy! Did we have guppies! But after a couple of months of saving and trading, we had enough tanks bubbling with angel fish and iridescents to short out most of the house.

On Saturdays throughout this first semester, Chris took the driver's training course and spent the time from 11:00 A.M. till 2:00 P.M. touring, at first the immediate vicinity, and later the freeways. He was really excited about getting his license.

Christmas of 1971 was fast approaching. We were determined to buy something that all the boys had wanted for a long time—a pool table. We had tried to manage it the year before, but found it too costly. Our objectives were to draw the family closer together, encourage young people to come around, and create a climate of lightness and laughter within our own walls. The pool table, therefore, was a unanimous decision. Shopping was left to Chris and me, and we enjoyed every minute of it. We toured every place in town, weighing coverings, slate, wood, size, and price. At long last, we zeroed in on a table at Montgomery Ward. The wood was simulated walnut, the bed thin slate over three-quarter-inch pressed wood, and the price, including four cues and heavily weighted balls, was just on target. We had a little more comparing to do, and it was almost a week later before we got back to place our order. The model was no longer in stock. Adversity was no news to us, so we persuaded the salesman (who called himself, "smiling Sam") to check with the warehouse. As luck would have it, they had just one left, but there was a question as to whether they could deliver it by

Christmas. I explained that the table *was* our Christmas, and Sam gave us his word that the pool table would be in our rumpus room before the turkey was on the table. As Christmas Eve dawned, the decorations were in place, the turkey was thawing on the sideboard, Bing Crosby's "White Christmas" was showing the wear of many seasons, and the rumpus room—long since having been measured and altered to accommodate the new arrival—stood ready. The rainy season had arrived early in Southern California and if a truck did turn in our cul-de-sac, we had difficulty reading the lettering on it through the downpour. Four o'clock arrived, a time when most businesses, having taken a tired accounting of disheveled stock and exhausted personnel, reluctantly close their doors. I glanced under our tree. There was one package: a small walnut rack which was to have held the cues. Presents weren't everything, we all knew that, but the thought that this might be Chris' last Christmas haunted me again, and I was sure I had made a dreadful mistake. Despite the terrible rain, and the darkness creeping over the Eve of Christmas, we kept up the jokes. Chris never doubted for a minute that "smiling Sam" would come through. Every few minutes, someone made a joke about hearing a truck. It was always followed by silence. It was Dad who finally shouted, "Here it is!" I was sitting in the living room and didn't even get up. Chris opened the kitchen door and a hoot rang out, followed by another and another. We all craned our necks out the back door as something huge and black and wet backed itself into our driveway. "Sam," I thought, "God bless you!"

There was just one man on the truck, and he, Bill, and the older boys had a devil of a time dragging the thing into the house. Even though the side yard was a sea of mud, it had to be brought around that way and through the rumpus room door. Nobody minded at all the fact that the blue carpet was covered with corrugated mush. We mixed a drink, gave Bing one more chance to enliven the spirit, and with directions spread all over the floor, set about the happy task of setting up the gift that would represent the last Christmas we were ever to enjoy together.

Since the gang considered the pool table as more of a man's gift, they surprised me with something special—a beautiful new steam iron, ironing board, and all the accessories. As Chris was always the official gift wrapper in the house, I cherish it all the more because he did a super job of camouflaging it and keeping it hidden for weeks. To this day, I never touch an iron to a pair of cords that I don't have a mental picture of that big surprise standing beside the tree, swathed in foil and covered with stick-on bows. That Christmas morning, when I was already overcome with emotion, Chris sprung another surprise. He had been drinking a goodly amount of tea over the past two years, so he presented me with a new "singing" tea kettle to make it more fun to prepare. And to warm my chapped hands on cold days in the nursery school playground, he accompanied the first surprise with a pair of warm woolen gloves. "Bright copper kettles, and warm woolen mittens," I thought. "These are a few of my favorite things." No, they are my most cherished possessions. Among my most cherished things, you will also find a hand-made sign which was scotch-taped to the outside of Chris' bedroom door every year. It reads, "Santa's Workshop—Keep Out!"

The older boys bought Chris a very large poster in black and white. The scene was a very barren hillside, punctuated by one lonely but very beautiful tree. The inscription read, "Let It Be." It occupied prime space over Chris' bed for a long time, and served to remind me of the contract I had vowed to fulfill.

The pool table turned out to be a wonderful choice. The older boys who had played on other tables around the neighborhood were instant pros. Mark and Kevin's friends came around in droves, lapping up Cokes and potato chips. Chris and his friends were there too, sometimes having to draw straws with the older boys to determine who would sit out a game. One night, while I was preparing dinner, I overheard one of Mark's twenty-year-old friends say something complimentary about Mark's shot. Another replied, "Oh yeah, if you think he's good, you should take on his little brother." I couldn't see it from the kitchen, but I could imagine that shy grin lighting up Chris' face.

OH, GOD! LET HIM LIVE A LITTLE!

In January 1972, another small success! After a visit to his surgeon, Chris was moved into the regular physical education class. He was delighted! The football season was over, and with track and swimming ahead, it seemed like a healthy maneuver, and one which would help to reinforce Chris' belief that he was, indeed, making steady progress. But each small success seemed to prefigure disappointment. The whole family was playing a sort of "run for your life" game, i.e., we wanted Chris to do everything and see everything possible in the short time he had left. A couple of weeks after Christmas, he received a good grade in Driver's Training, and, after just a few short spins around the neighborhood, I encouraged him to take his test. Driving is something that all young men look forward to and I didn't want him to miss it.

He was "riding the crest" the day we went down to the Motor Vehicle Bureau to take the test, but though he received a 100% grade on the written test, he was obviously nervous. I had been to this place many times, both in taking the test myself, and with the older boys. We decided that we should run around the course a time or two, to gain confidence. When Chris and the inspector pulled away for the test drive I may have prayed harder than I did in the waiting room at U.C.L.A. on that fateful day. But what I thought would be five minutes stretched into fifteen, and I felt a great sense of relief when the old Falcon slid into the back parking lot and pulled up beside me. I checked the expressions of their faces. Chris looked serene. The inspector, I decided, looked satisfied. He was carefully making marks on the clipboard in his lap. A few words began to filter out through the open window: "... overly cautious ... full stop. ..." The door on the inspector's side opened and he beckoned to me. I noticed the clipboard in his lap; it was a maze of red markings. Chris was vehemently defending himself. "Is there anything wrong with being overly cautious?" I heard him yell. As the inspector got out of the car, one sentence burned itself into my mind, "We'll see this young man in a couple of weeks." My heart felt like lead as I got into the car and pulled out of the driveway. Chris was furious and fighting back tears. For blocks, he pounded on the seat and maintained he hadn't made a single error. It doesn't matter now. He was defeated, and never got a chance to try again.

Sometime in late January 1972, I happened to pass his bedroom to catch him putting himself through the standard neurological tests. Each time he closed his eyes, he lost his balance and fell against the bed. I knew that he was aware of a regression, and although I didn't want to admit it, even to Bill, I had noticed it, too. He was tiring more easily and vomiting more frequently. I wanted more than anything to believe the surgeon's latest prognosis, but something told me it was overly optimistic.

As Bill began noticing the deterioration in Chris' condition, I nagged all the more for him to attend one of Kathryn Kuhlman's miracle services at the Shrine Auditorium. I can't say if it was just because he was tired of hearing my voice, or because panic was growing within him, but he agreed. With the other boys standing by, and with all the food cooked and ready for the entire day, Dad and I took off, telling Chris we were going to a company cocktail party.

My luck ran out before the doors opened at the Shrine. We were packed shoulder to shoulder in the waiting crowd. A man just behind Bill, who sang most loudly for the entire three hours we waited, kept trying to get Bill to join in. I thought at times that Bill might take a poke at him if he didn't shut up. Bill lasted the three hours, and we got seats inside, but the emotionalism, Miss Kuhlman's prancing around the stage, and the theatrical atmosphere were too much for him. In spite of my pleadings, he left and waited for me in the car. The service usually lasts until around 5:00 P.M., but I felt uneasy and came away at three. He was silent all the way home, but Chris' worsened condition motivated him to attend one more time.

I learned that it was possible to buy a seat on a chartered bus going to the Shrine Auditorium. The bus was jammed, and Bill was surprised to find that there were even people at the boarding point on a stand-by list. The advantage of taking the bus was that the passengers from some twenty or thirty busses were admitted to the auditorium first. As we disembarked from the bus, a young Mexican girl just ahead of us was having a terrible time trying to handle a baby, many bundles (probably containing lunch and diapers), and at the same time, help a very elderly, ailing woman, who might have been her mother. So, Bill offered to hold the baby for her until they got settled on the sidewalk. The baby was darling, but when he handed it back, his new suit was wet from the elbow to the knee. The look on his face was so priceless that I laughed till I cried. Once inside the auditorium, he had no choice but to stay to the end of the service, since we were taking the bus back home. Something touched him deeply that day, and before the services were over, he was wiping tears from his eyes.

I recall Bill saying to me once that if I ever took Chris to one of those services, he'd leave me. Another time, toward the very end, he asked me, "What are you going to think of Kathryn Kuhlman if Chris dies?" I answered with conviction, "No matter which way it goes, I know I've seen miracles."

Around the middle of February, I decided that no miracle was going to happen at home. I decided to take Chris to a service. The fact that we had so long kept his condition from him made the excursion nearly impossible. Mark and Kevin were helpful in a most roundabout way. After long months of prayer, they had almost ceased to believe in anything. Neither went to church. They felt either that God was not there or that He had abandoned us. I honestly can't say that I blamed them for their feelings. We had all been through almost four years of real agony, praying together in secret, having Masses said for Chris, and making our private novenas. Nerves were on edge, meals were out of focus, and a good night's sleep was only a dream. All of this came at a time, for them, when manhood threatened to replace childhood, the military draft was snapping at their heels, and college studies demanded serious concentration. God love them! They both made a valiant effort, and I applaud them for sticking with it and not copping out when the going got tough. This would have been a perfect excuse for a boy of less moral fiber to find his way to narcotics, run away from home, or let his grades go to the devil. But not our sons, thank God, not our sons.

I began to set the stage for our trip to the Shrine Auditorium weeks in advance. One Sunday morning, in Chris' presence, I "accidentally" stumbled over Kathryn Kuhlman's telecast, making no bones about my amazement over the possibilities of modern-day miracles. We talked about the miracles in the Bible, and agreed that it would, indeed, be unlikely that God would allow great numbers of miracles in Biblical times and few in modern times. (Incidentally, I had given a great deal of tearful thought to taking him to Lourdes, but the budget just wouldn't stand it. I thought of borrowing the money, and just getting on a plane, but I was stopped there by the fact that Chris would have to know the whole truth. And what if there was no miracle!)

After watching Kathryn Kuhlman's telecasts with Chris several Sundays, I asked him what he thought of taking his troublesome stomach up to the Shrine and, while there, tossing in a prayer or two that Mark and Kev would return to the church. He reluctantly agreed. Bill did too. Now, there remained only one detail to be worked out—how to get him in without a wait. He never could have weathered it. Somewhere back in my mind, I recalled seeing on one of the telecasts, a woman who held a high position in one of our local high schools. She had been cured of a lingering illness, and now in gratitude she served as an usher at the auditorium when Miss Kuhlman was in town. I called her at her office, and I will always be grateful to her, because, without ever having met us, she was instantly ready to help. She agreed to let us in through the side door, and to make no mention of the nature of Chris' illness.

Our whole family tried to make an adventure of it, each, of course, never letting on that he had been there before. Only Chris and I were going, but it took the whole crew to pack us off. Chris was noticeably impressed by the long lines of wheel chairs and stretchers as we neared the side door. I recognized our kind friend at once from her appearance on television, and we were whisked through the door and handed over to an usher without incident.

The Shrine is a huge place, with balconies

reaching up three or four stories. Since childhood, Chris had always had a fear of heights. (I remember a baseball game at Anaheim Stadium, and the fear he experienced in climbing to our seat in the second to last row.) Now, with his coordination a little less than normal, he found it doubly difficult to climb to the third-level balcony. He hung onto me and to the ends of each seat for dear life. We found a seat next to the extreme right-hand wall, and right on top of an exit, which gave him some sense of security.

The stage seemed a mile away, but the scene was one of pure beauty. Two concert grand pianos occupied prime positions. Behind these, and up on risers stretching the full width of the stage, a tremendously large, all-volunteer choir, dressed in brilliant colors, and under the baton of a most accomplished director, entertained the audience until every seat was filled. On stage, just in front of the choir, was a section reserved for dignitaries: rabbis and ministers, priests and nuns, and doctors from around the world. Wheel chairs occupied the once-fashionable "boxes" on the one side, while on the other, a section of the lower balcony was reserved for the deaf, to whom every word of the service was communicated through sign language.

Many in the great body of the audience, I'm sure, were there for a healing, but I am sure as many more attended just to enjoy the spectacle. I felt something there that I have never felt in any single church: a oneness. Everyone cares, everyone is helping everyone else: the sick and the well, the blacks and the whites, the old and the young. "Notice the Christians—how they love one another." It is beautiful to behold, and makes one realize that religion is not in a certain church, on a certain corner, but, rather, in that great cathedral —the temple of the Holy Spirit—one's self.

The music built to a great crescendo, the audience rose to its feet, and Kathryn Kuhlman emerged from the wings and took her place at center stage. On this particular day, she began by centering her attention on the young people in the audience. After a short message, she asked all the young who wanted Jesus to come into their lives, to come up on stage. You can imagine my surprise and apprehension when, without a word, Chris got up and started down the many steep flights of stairs. He disappeared through an exit on the third balcony, and it seemed like an eternity before he reappeared far below, making his way up one of the main aisles toward the stage. There were throngs of young people, and Chris squeezed into a position on the extreme right-hand side of the stage. I was holding my breath, almost afraid to pray, as Miss Kuhlman made her way across the stage, touching each young face. She almost reached Chris—but not quite—before she turned, blessed the whole assembly, and dismissed them.

We stayed as late as we could. There were many beautiful miracles that day, but Chris was not one of them.

6

Good Night, Mr. Christopher

Two years had elapsed since Grandpa and Grandma had left Chris at U.C.L.A. Hospital and returned to Rochester. Now, with spring in the air, they were coming back to California to check on his progress. They were surprised at his great crop of hair. It was long now, and hid not only the scars, but that ugly shunt behind his ear.

Things had not been going well with Chris. He was experiencing deterioration in balance, intermittent double vision, and increased vomiting. On a recent check-up with the surgeon, Chris asked, "What's that thing behind my ear?" (I had been telling him I thought it was a calcium deposit on the bone.) The doctor answered, calmly, "A tube." Sitting there in my corner of the examining room, my knees turned to water. "Here it comes," I thought. I knew the surgeon had never agreed with our decision to keep the truth from Chris. But it didn't. Chris didn't say a word. I kept wondering what I was going to say when he hit me with a hundred questions on the way home, but, completely out of tune with his inquisitive nature, he never did that either. I felt sure that the doctors had just confirmed what Chris had suspected all along.

Apparently, the doctor could see no drastic change in Chris' condition, but he did recommend that we see an ophthalmologist at U.C.L.A. to determine what might be done about the double vision. Please don't ever try to tell me that the personality of a medical man is of little consequence, for the unbelievable diplomacy with which this wonderful man handled Chris will negate all of your arguments. He talked baseball while putting Chris through a battery of tests and X-rays. Then, treating him almost as an equal, he complimented Chris on his choice of surgeons and on his remarkable recovery. Congratulating Chris on his 20-20 vision, and with an encouraging word to "hang in there," he dismissed us with a prescription for a mild tranquilizer which would probably clear up Chris' "temporary problem." I found out later that his report to the surgeon was quite different. It took a big man to do what he did.

I've always been a dreamer, I guess, and now more than ever I clung to every little sign, every little hope. I felt so close to God in these days that I considered anything in the least out of the ordinary a personal message from the Almighty. One evening I was ironing and watching on TV one of my favorite musicals, "Brigadoon." The very last line in the play is something to the effect that, "If you love someone enough, anything is possible, even a miracle!" I broke into tears again, and said to God, "You wouldn't fool me, would you?" Again, I thought He said, "No, don't worry." I believed Him.

In spring of '72, even though Grandpa was here, we followed the same routine: driving Chris to school, catching Kathryn Kuhlman, attending church, working at nursery school, and picking up Chris at noon. But now, instead of waiting for him while he kidded around with his friends, I found that he was always waiting for me. I can see him still, sitting on a little rock wall outside the locker room, a sickly expression where the smile used to be.

One morning, he woke up complaining that his left hand felt "funny," the fingers numb. I panicked, but said that he had probably slept on it. He didn't mention it again for a couple of days. Then, he said, "What's the matter with my arm? It won't do what I want it to do." He was a "lefty" and began having a problem with writing. I suggested an in-between visit to the doctor, but Chris flatly refused.

We made one more triumphant visit to Disneyland—Chris, Bill, and I, and two of Chris' friends. Apprehension filled me when we bought their tickets at the gate and made a date to meet the boys back there at midnight. He was just a little rocky, and though he had a little money to treat his friends, I knew he himself couldn't eat. We ran into them around eleven o'clock while waiting in line at the America the Beautiful pavilion. I had never been there before and neither had Chris. I can only describe it as a movie in the round. The viewer stands in the middle of a large room, holding onto a railing, while a movie completely surrounds him, giving the impression that he is a part of the action. We rode a fire-truck, crazily, down the steets of San Francisco, did a flip in a plane, rose and fell with the high seas. It was fantastic! I looked at Chris; he was ashen. There was no apparent way out, so he closed his eyes until it was over. As soon as he got his "sea legs" back, however, he finished the evening as though nothing had happened. In fact, his friends never knew that anything had.

On Easter Sunday, 1972, the whole family, along with Grandpa and Grandma, were scheduled to get together for dinner with our relatives in Santa Monica. Chris awakened that morning with a touch of flu, accompanied by body aches and a low-grade fever. Since we saw Grandpa and Grandma so seldom the affair was special, and they were all so disappointed when we decided to keep Chris home. Because the little reunion would have shrunk to just five people without them, Bill and the boys went without us.

Chris spent the day in bed, reading and

watching television. Though we kept up the usual aspirin, fluids, and rest routine, he became steadily worse. His fever continued to rise, though I sponged him all afternoon. By five o'clock it reached a hundred and five, and he complained of a bad headache and sore throat. I called Bill and he and the boys came right home. In the evening, we reached a doctor and, through a local hospital's pharmacy, obtained the necessary antibiotics to lick the fever. However, either the particular strain of flu or the high fever surely must have accelerated the growth of that awful tumor, for the dear boy went steadily downhill from that moment.

Two weeks before Memorial Day, when he was feeling a little stronger, we thought the warm sun and a change of scenery would be good for him. We stretched the budget one more time and took a long weekend in Palm Springs. Through the services of a travel agency, we were lucky to find a beautiful spot in Palm Desert, a combination tennis club and country club, with sprawling green lawns, sparkling pools, and exotic restaurants. We had rarely seen real desert before, and so taken was Chris with the velvet whiteness of the surroundings that he insisted on getting out of the car and putting his footprints in the sand. I often wonder how long they remained before a silent wind wiped them away.

He made a valiant effort to enjoy himself, though it was too obviously an effort. He couldn't get out of bed until noon, so we brought his meals up on a tray and he enjoyed them on a delightful balcony directly overlooking the pool. On two afternoons, he got into his trunks and went for a swim. His beautiful crawl never gave away the fact that his left arm was misbehaving. Once or twice, he even ventured to dive off the board, but I feel sure that this was done for no other reason than to reassure us. On a couple of occasions I saw him standing off to one side, alone, under a big tree, taking a long look at the players on the tennis courts, or watching an older boy doing somersaults off the high board. Dear God! I hoped he wasn't thinking what we were thinking.

On the last night there, we tried a big dinner in the dining room. Purposely, we went in late. There was a tennis banquet in an adjoining room and we listened to the laughter and applause. The dining room was deserted except for ourselves. It was beautifully appointed, quiet and cool. He decided to try that lobster I owed him. About halfway through it, he made a desperate dash from the room, with me close on his heels, and vomited miserably in the bushes out in back by the trash cans. "Oh, Lord!" I thought bitterly, "where in hell are you?"

Chris never got back to school, nor did I. His eyes were jigging in his head again, his arm was nearly useless, he was thin and exhausted. We were so tired and so scared, we were beginning to wonder whether or not we could see it through and let him die at home as we had planned. He hated those hospitals so much!

The family next door was away a good part of

the time, and they loaned me a key to their door so I could use their phone out of earshot of Chris. By now, I was making panic calls to all the doctors, all the prayer groups and most of the faith healers in the country. The good doctors at U.C.L.A., meanwhile, were contacting medical centers around the country looking for a last-resort measure. They decided that more cobalt was impractical, and chemotherapy was ruled out too.

A friend called one day to tell me about a doctor in Mexico who was having great success with a new drug called Laetrile. I understood that Stanford Medical Center was experimenting with it, so I called from the phone next door. They denied ever having heard of the drug. Through his job, Bill knew some people at Stanford and contacted them. A day or two later, we got a report back. Yes, they had been experimenting with the drug, but not only did they consider the drug completely without merit, it was against the law to use it in this country. By this time, however, I'd heard other reports of the drug's almost miraculous effects, and I decided to call the doctor in Mexico. He was most gracious over the phone, but informed me that the drug had never been used on brain cancer. He suggested that they might, for the very first time, try injecting it directly into the spinal fluid. We were afraid the effects could be worse than what he was suffering now. Still the name of that drug was appearing in medical journals and newspapers with increasing frequency. I learned one day that at a

103

large Los Angeles hotel there was a convention, the purpose of which was to discuss the pros and cons of using Laetrile in this country. I was truly desperate now, and decided to drive to Mexico and talk to the doctor myself. However, Chris needed me here, so Dad and Kev drove down early one Saturday morning. They told Chris they were going up to look over the campus at U.C., Santa Barbara, the university Kevin would attend in the fall. When they drove back into the garage that night, they were both shaking their heads—no.

Memorial Day weekend, 1972, found Chris sicker than ever, and the family about as low in spirit as can be imagined. Bill and I had a crying conference in the garage, and decided that we were insulting the boy's intelligence and had better tell him. Bill went up to his room first, and, as I listened at the foot of the stairs, I heard him hint to Chris that, just perhaps, that tumor was showing some activity again. Chris was instantly on the defensive. The tumor was gone, and he didn't want to hear any more about it. Poor darling, no wonder, after what he'd been through! I also tried to give him an opportunity to talk about it or to ask questions. No dice! The subject was closed. On Mothers' Day, I talked with the surgeon by phone. There had been many meetings between the radiologists and himself, and they could come up with nothing. He ventured a guess that Chris had about two months to live and suggested that we either put him in a hospital or keep him home and give him nursing care.

My birthday, June 9, arrived and nothing could dissuade Chris from getting out of bed and going to the Peninsula Center to buy a gift. How he could think of me at a time like that, I'll never know, but no amount of pleading would change his mind. He was so weak, and I was so concerned about his falling, that I insisted on going along. He wouldn't hear of it, so Kevin got one of his good friends to accompany them and help Chris walk. I cried all the time they were gone, and I cry now whenever I think of it. But Kev assured me that Chris really enjoyed himself, and that they had many a laugh over what Chris considered Kev's poor taste in handbags. I have the lovely one which Chris selected; I will have it until the day I die.

He left the house just once more, and that was during the same week. We were still trying to find ways to amuse him and brighten his days. His double vision was so bad that he could no longer enjoy television, though we had it on a good part of the time just for company. Mark (through his own resources) had just bought a tape-deck for his car, and Chris, though he had never seen it, was very much taken with the idea. Bill agreed that it would be a great idea to get him stereo components for his room. When we told Chris about it, he said he didn't want it because he knew we couldn't afford it. We lied about having had a recent insurance dividend, and after making a half dozen calls, comparing prices and features, we charged up a beauty at Sears. He insisted on coming along to see it before buying. (After all, what would a mother know about components?) It was an awful effort for him to get into a pair of shorts and a shirt, but he made it! We toured the parking lot at Sears for a long time before finding a spot right in front of the door. He was so rocky that he needed support all the way, and we had to stop in the furniture department to rest. As I've mentioned before, Chris was always concerned about everyone except himself. His face told me at once the set he liked best, but he was worried about the price. After much friendly arguing, and my repeated assurance that, after all, it would be enjoyed by the whole family, we consummated the deal. Back in the car he was ecstatic. They couldn't deliver it for a week. That gave us a few more tomorrows.

June exams were over now. Mark and a friend had made elaborate plans for a trip around the country in the summer. He was ready to call it off for Chris' sake, but he had been through the wringer that year, and we encouraged him to keep his plans, leaving us his itinerary so we could notify him in case of emergency. Mark left in the middle of June, with a packed car and a lot of apprehensions.

As sick as he was, Chris was still fun to be with. He never complained about his problems; he made light of them. His double vision, for instance. Once when I was standing in the doorway of his room asking him whether or not he thought I should go down to the kitchen and rustle up some lunch, he laughed and quipped, "Why don't one of you go and the other stay here?"

Then there was the Saturday when he implored me to get his pants and take him to church. In our Catholic Church, it is mandatory for everyone to go to confession and receive communion between the first Sunday of Lent and Trinity Sunday. He must have heard one of us mention that the next day was Trinity Sunday, and he realized he had not received the sacraments. I sat down on his bed and explained that since he had never missed communion as long as he could walk, he was surely a little saint in God's eyes. But he wouldn't buy it. "For heaven's sake," he begged, "don't get me excommunicated!" Nothing would do but that I would call the priest and get his official opinion. The priest generously offered to come to the house with the sacraments, but made it quite clear that it was not at all necessary. (He and I knew that Chris had received the last rites of the church many times.) When I told Chris what the priest had said, his face relaxed, his mind was at ease.

Something very special came in the mail around the middle of June. It was a huge card, the front displaying a picture of a most adorable, but slightly pathetic little guy. On the inside was a message that meant more to Chris than anything since Vicki. It read: "Dear Chris, Your second period Geometry class has decided by unanimous agreement, and I concur, that tests are not the only measure of scholarship. Sincerity and effort play an equal role, and besides, most of your grades this year have been A's. So, by our first unanimous agreement in months, Chris, you're excused from the final exam and your grade in the course is an A. We all wish you the very best. Very Sincerely, Your Geometry Class." This was followed by the signatures of twenty-seven students, along with that of Chris' teacher, Mr. Neil Ward, and his sophomore counselor.

Chris broke down and cried when he read it. We had a terrible time trying to settle on a method of acknowledgment. By now, he couldn't write at all, he could hardly move. He didn't want me to write a note for him; he was too proud. Finally we decided that a telegram would be just the ticket. The wire went something like this: "I want you to know how very much I appreciate your kind thoughts, not to speak of the A grade. After much deliberation, and in all good conscience, I must say that I also concur. I will be back in the fall, and support your confidence by proving that I can earn that grade in the next semester. Sincerely, Chris." It wasn't until many months later that I discovered that the telegram was never delivered.

Chris' infirmities were emphasized now by the fact that the other kids were out of school. Mark and his friend were off on their trip, and Kev was working at Marineland. As Chris lay almost motionless in our king-sized bed, he could hear kids splashing in their pools, riding their mini-bikes up and down the street, and running with dime in hand to meet the ice-cream man. Once, he said, sadly, "What a way to spend a summer vacation." "What a way," I thought, "to spend the last four years of a very short lifetime."

Then one quiet morning, it hit. It was the penance we had to pay for playing it our own way and trying to spare him the truth. I won't name the early morning, Los Angeles television show we never missed watching. Chris and I were watching because it was light and cheerful and usually started our day on a happy note, covering in small but interesting shorts, the gamut from sports to theater, from international affairs to human interest. That particular morning, I was feeding Chris his breakfast, and they were on "human interest," discussing the case of a pathetic little girl who was desperately ill. Before I could gracefully flip to another channel it came out, two sentences run together as though no punctuation separated them: "Does she know she's terminal, that she's going to die?" I froze in my chair. I was caught in my own trap and could think of no way to rationalize my own way out. The words faltered as I put the ice-tea straw into his mouth. I had never forgotten that night in the hospital, and I knew that he hadn't either. Another bite of breakfast. They had switched to another subject. Then the words came quietly and undisturbed. "Mom, you're a good woman." If I hadn't had so much practice at hiding emotions, I surely would have cried. But I just hugged him and said, "Thanks. And you're the greatest kid in the world." From that moment, though I think it happened a long time before, we were one. He knew that we knew, that he knew. It was as simple as that.

In those days, his faith in God and in us was something to witness. He never asked a question. He knew that he was loved beyond life itself, and I'm sure he was satisfied in his heart that we had done everything possible. His voice was only a whisper now, and on a few occasions when we left his room, he would say, "Will you turn off the television, please? I want to think awhile." During many of these quiet times, Bill would sit on the bed, holding Chris' head in both of his hands, an expression of unbelievable tenderness on his face.

At the suggestion of his surgeon, we had enlisted the services of a local doctor to see Chris through to the end. I often thought at the time how unfair it was to lean on this good man, since he saw only the worst and could do nothing. But he was most kind in making frequent house calls. The first time he visited, Chris joked, "I must be dying. It's the only thing that would bring a doctor out on a house call." But the doctor was a gem and continued to bolster the boy's morale in every way possible.

On the first day of July, 1972, Chris was clearly near the end. Dad and Kev were at work, and Kev's girl friend, Janice, kept the vigil with me. Our poor, brave little friend was breathing most laboriously, and he was hallucinating at times. The doctor had been there the evening before and found Chris' lungs clear and his vital signs still strong. But he was so much worse that day I called Bill at the office and Kev at Marineland. It seemed as if they were here immediately. Bill took one glance at Chris and called an ambulance. Kev and I were horrified! We had made an agreement to let Chris die at home. Even as they slid the stretcher into the ambulance in front of the house, Kev and I were begging Dad to change his mind. He wouldn't budge. I occupied the front seat beside the driver, while Kev and Dad followed along behind in our car. I remember being astounded at the roughness of the ride! Sitting backwards in the front seat, I held his little head in both hands to keep it from bobbing around. We might as well have been riding a buckboard.

The hospital had everything ready for our arrival. The good doctor who had been attending Chris was out of town, and we hurriedly shook hands with a stand-in—a man who within the next hour gained our deepest respect.

Where one finds such presence of mind in a crisis like this, I will never know, but we remembered before leaving the house to make up a large index card, printed in bold felt pen. It read, "DON'T MENTION CANCER. HE DOESN'T KNOW." I showed this to every nurse and doctor who entered the door of his room. After X-rays they immediately placed him in a cold, wet tent. A saline bottle was hung over his bed and hooked up to correct dehydration —a condition we didn't even suspect. Two hours later, he sat up in bed and asked in a bewildered voice touched with anger, "How the devil did I get here?" Shortly, the verdict came back: double pneumonia. I was never so relieved in my life, and we both (Kev and I) thanked Bill for his insight and quick-thinking. Double pneumonia was nothing to fool with, but it put us many rungs up the ladder from death.

The doctor told Chris that he would be out in four days, but the four stretched to eight. I was allowed to stay with Chris the whole week. Many a cup of hot tea or glass of iced tea was brewed in the little kitchenette next to his room.

July 4 came during that week, and served to bring back stinging memories of block parties and picnic tables covered with American flags. Chris was well enough by then to take a wheel chair ride down to the end of the hall where a large picture window took in some of the community fireworks displays. But he had no heart for it. We swung his bed facing the windows in his room and made an effort to interest him in the Roman candles bursting over Malaga Cove. Still, his thoughts were elsewhere, and the Fourth passed with his having lost any feeling he ever had of independence.

I left him with Bill and Kev one day and ran over to the Broadway, looking for a gift that might bring back that smile we all cherished. I scooped up several pairs of pajamas and a karate bathrobe.

Then, as though God were fulfilling some master plan, it hit me! The lobster and the $68.00 had long since been repaid, but the "Let It Be" album still remained on the slate. I decided that a tape for his new stereo might please him more than the record, and was lucky enough to find one. He was just delighted, and though he couldn't play it in the hospital, or even roll over to look at it, he asked us several times a day to reassure him that it was sitting right beside him on the bedside table.

The "Let It Be" tape seemed to make him happy enough to show his sense of humor once more. Many times a day, he was put on breathing machines to clear up the mucus in his lungs. One of the technicians asked one day, "Hey, Chris, how long did it take you to grow that mustache?" It still amounted to nothing more than a shadow of peach fuzz, but without hesitating a moment, Chris, with an absolutely straight face answered, "Four years." Everyone laughed, of course, and the peach fuzz spread into a grin.

His homecoming was again happy, happier than I can ever tell you. He was coming home to die, we all knew that, but still, there was a glorious feeling of seeing it through together, and a triumphant awareness of doing it his way. We had a new Toyota now, and, with the front seat tilted almost to a prone position, he lay there humming his favorite songs all the way home, his foot tapping out the beat on the floor mat.

Our big bed was ready to welcome Chris when

113

he came home, but he wanted to be back in his own room with his stereo. He seemed quite bright and cheerful sitting up in his own bed with the Beatles setting the mood. But we had been warned that the lungs would fill up again, and would eventually take him. Our own doctor was back now, and had been in touch with the surgeon at U.C.L.A. We were told that, in X-raying his chest, they had discovered a new tumor on his left rib—undoubtedly the cause of the paralysis in the left arm. Once again, the possibility of radiation in this new area was discussed at length, and dismissed as impractical.

During this interval, we were always in touch with Mark by phone, and, though he was quite disturbed by Chris' hospitalization, we encouraged him to finish out his trip, since nothing more could be done here. We promised to keep in touch daily.

A day or two after Chris came home, we had one last happy time. The doorbell rang one afternoon, and a group of his friends hesitantly asked if they could come in and see him. As luck would have it, he was sitting up in bed, dressed in new pajamas, and feeling quite chipper. The kids had never seen his new stereo components, and this gave Chris an opportunity to feel quite important as they made a great fuss over him. They brought their dog, too, a big male collie, and as Vicki was in heat at the time, the party became lively without any provocation. The kids played "Risk" on the floor of Chris' room, the dogs raced around the house, and the Beatles tied the whole thing to-gether. I was both crying and laughing as I peeled potatoes for dinner.

The hospital provided a follow-up service for patients who went home in Chris' condition, and it was not long before we had occasion to take advantage of it. Because it was getting increasingly difficult for him to sit up and to get up to the bathroom, we rented an electric hospital bed. Bill and I were deeply sad as we carted Chris' own little bed downstairs to be stored on the rafters in the garage, but we were making room for the rented bed which was to be delivered that afternoon. We moved Chris into our room during the transition. When it was delivered, we talked in loud voices about wanting to rent it only for a week, while our son recovered from pneumonia. After it was set up, we all took turns jumping in, pushing buttons, and laughing at what fun it was, but Chris would have nothing to do with it. He never left our bedroom from that day on.

During those last two weeks, I slept with Chris, and Bill slept in the hospital bed. Mark came home full of great tales about the night clubs in New Orleans, sunsets over the desert, and a round of good times with Grandpa in Rochester, New York. It was a lift we all needed, and we made the very most of it, begging him time and again to "tell us more."

By now, Chris was so uncomfortable that even the sheets on the bed hurt his tender skin. Each time he got up to go to the bathroom (a procedure upon which he absolutely insisted), we saw a look, not only of pain, but of sheer panic on his face. We rented an air mattress, an electrically operated sheet of plastic bubbles which alternately inflate and deflate, easing the pressure and strain on different parts of the body. When we brought it up to his room, he whispered to me, "Mom, is this a prelude to anything?" "You bet it is," I said. "It's a prelude to a good night's sleep." It was, too. It so comforted his exhausted frame that he slept a full eight hours, right in the middle of the day.

Toward the end of July, 1972, a hot spell engulfed us. Temperatures soared into the high nineties, and we decided to buy a large fan just to keep the air moving in that room. As it turned out, a neighbor was good enough to loan us just what we needed. The heat hung around most of the night. Because the sliding glass door leading to the balcony opened from the side, we got in the habit of tucking the drapes back and hooking them around the door handle. From our vantage point in bed, Chris and I watched the stars, and many times reminisced about other times and other places, far into the night. We walked again through the woods in Livingston, traversed the whole of Disneyland, tobogganed in the snows of New Jersey, and revisited the candy shop at Lake Arrowhead. I knew he was scared, and he knew we were broken-hearted, but never a word of this passed between us. Sometimes, when silence interrupted us, I'd ask,

"What are you thinking about?" He'd always reply, "I'm just looking out at my little piece of sky."

One night I fell asleep on the couch from sheer exhaustion, and the family, not wishing to wake me, decided that Kev should stay with Chris. I'll never know what transpired that night, but Kev tells me it was a wonderful night. They were close in age, of course, and had always been real buddies; Kev had taught Chris in better days how to ride a bike, how to master a skate board, and, in short, just about everything he needed to know in the way of being a boy. I guess they hashed over a lifetime —be it ever so short—in language that only boys could understand. I am so grateful that they had those last moments together. Mark shared many sweet moments with Chris, too. I think that he always felt a pang of conscience over having taken that trip. But he shouldn't have, for Mark was always the most unselfish one of us all. He was the one who did more dishes, vacuumed more carpets, and willingly spent hour upon hour making Chris comfortable.

In the quiet heat of August 2, 1972, his last day crept in—like a summer storm that you know is coming, but never expect to arrive. The borrowed fan was moving the curtains ever so slightly as I brought up "Phase I" of his breakfast. He found it easier to eat little bits at a time, and this was a dish of cold cantaloupe, cut into very small pieces. He couldn't move at all now, and his back was towards me as I entered the room. For the past few days, we had not been able to tell whether or not he was still with us, until we saw his fingers lift ever so slightly in an effort to wave. I was surprised and delighted to find him, on this particular morning, quite alert, and eager for conversation. It took about a half hour of laborious effort to get down the melon. I read aloud the morning paper, starting as always with his favorite section, the sports page. At this slow pace, the meals went on all day, really, with a rest between each course. I washed my hair and set it—a real treat! Then, I brought up the cream of wheat. This went down well too, and I was pleased.

Mark and Kev were home that day, and as had become the practice, we spent every moment in Chris' room. Just after lunch, I noticed that his pulse rate had quickened. I could see it beating furiously in his neck. He began talking in rather a thick whisper and I had to put my ear close to his mouth to make out what he was saying. He spoke of Kev and himself bombing ships in a creek, and of a game of hockey played with brooms. He was hallucinating again, I was sure, and I called Bill. He came home at once, and with tears in his eyes, saw what I had seen earlier, that at intervals Chris' hands and mouth turned black. It was terrifying.

I do not recall the balance of that day vividly. The doctor was summoned in the afternoon, and he did his best to prepare us. I recall that Bill and I had a talk in the backyard sometime around the dinner hour. We knew that this was the end, and agreed that it was going to be a long night. Mark had been asked to come into work at Hughes Market, from 4:30 to 9:30 P.M. He didn't want to go, but we encouraged him to get out of the house for a few hours, as we were certain we had many hours in which to keep the vigil.

At 9:15 P.M., Dad ran a short errand to the drugstore, just five minutes away. Kev and I were alone with Chris in the room, Kev on one side of the bed, myself on the other. Chris began to have great difficulty with his breathing. His lungs were full, we knew, and sometimes a change of position helped him to cough, relieving him somewhat. I suggested to Kev that we try to turn him over. Ever so gently, we began to roll him. Just as we did Chris' eyes fixed. He was gone. I sat stupified as Kev said, "Good-bye, little buddy."

Sirens blared, lights flashed, the voices of friends and strangers rose and fell. It was blurred, in spite of all the warnings, by complete disbelief. We remembered at 9:30 that Mark would be getting off work, and we didn't want him to come upon that terrible scene without some preparation. One of our good neighbors drove out and met him around the corner to prepare him for the shock.

Shortly after Chris died, a priest from our church visited. None of the priests we knew well were on hand that night. This man was a stranger. He stood looking down at Chris and began talking to us about God's love. I screamed at him, "And where is God now?" I am ashamed that I couldn't receive his condolences with more dignity. I wish I could have been like Dad, steady and in complete control.

But underlying it all we knew that Chris had met his greatest challenge with the utmost dignity. He had done it his way. That was all that mattered. It was well after midnight before they came to take Chris away. We stood by the front door as they brought him down the stairs, swathed in a white sheet, looking like Lazarus coming forth from the tomb. I uncovered his face. I couldn't bear to see him that way.

At 3:00 A.M., when everyone else had finally left, the four of us sat around the living room as if we were made of stone. We had an appointment with the mortuary the next morning at ten o'clock, so Dad suggested we had better try to get some sleep. I was the first one in bed. Dad, Mark, and Kev roamed around aimlessly. I reached for the rosary on the night table as I had done just about every night of my life. Purely out of habit, I kissed the cross and began, "I believe in God, the Father Almighty . . . " Then I remembered that I had nothing left to pray for. I stared at the rosary. It looked like a string of dime-store beads. "How," I thought, "could the Blessed Lady let us down so miserably?" I clenched the rosary in my fist and hurled it across the room. It hit the mirror with a crash and slid down behind the dresser. Dad and Kev moved the dresser and handed the rosary back to me. I cried bitterly as I remembered that she, too, had lost a Son. May God forgive me.

We laid Chris on a green hill overlooking the Palos Verdes Peninsula, under a big tree closely resembling the "Let It Be" tree on his beloved poster. His little plot has an unlimited view of Los Angeles harbor (Harbor of the Angels) and ironically, of the Terminal Island Bridge. Vicki and I visit him every day, and the boys and Dad, on the weekends.

Though I know, if God is real, that Chris is not truly there, I still find peace in thinking of him sleeping there in his blue V-necked sweater and blue cords, his furry mustache above the smile we'll never forget. His "Let It Be" tape sleeps with him, along with a little shoe box we found on his closet shelf. Reminiscent of "The Littlest Angel," it contained his most precious possessions: seven decorative icicles, one for each Christmas tree we shared in this house; five little bags of rock candy from Lake Arrowhead; Vicki's ribbons and trophies; a few ribbons which Chris himself had won in the broadjump.

Chris' marker is plain except for a rosary which encircles it. I wanted to tell "her" I still believe. Bill chose the wording:

CHRISTOPHER T. MC IVERS
SO YOUNG—SO BRAVE—SO LOVED
1955–1972

From our vantage-point on the hill, Vicki and I

can hear the tinkling tune of the ice-cream man on the opposite hill, the cheers of Little Leaguers on an adjacent field, and the chimes of the beautiful bell-tower tolling the hour, no longer of any consequence to our dear Chris.

More than two years have elapsed since then, but even now, on a warm California night, when I lie nearly in the center of our king-sized bed, sleepless, still, and heavy with defeat, I look out at his "little piece of sky," and remember when we held his hand, and watched him die.

AFTERWORD

As an afterword, I have asked my family to answer the question I threw at the priest on the night of Chris' death:

WHERE IS GOD NOW?

FROM BILL:

Dear Chris:

Before your illness and death in 1972, I believed strongly in the idea of a "larger force," a "presence," a God which went much beyond the intellectual ability of any one of us to really comprehend, and I believe that none of us lived by bread alone, that somehow we all needed a spiritual nourishment and companionship during our existence to make life understandable and purposeful. I had always felt a companionship with God, as I know you did.

How do I feel now? My concept of a God, of the need of mankind for a God, of the need of all men for spiritual nourishment is essentially unchanged. But I feel that personally I have lost a sense of brotherhood, of companionship, of communication with God. As I think back on the whole ordeal, what comes through clearest to me now was your strength and calmness. I never heard you cry in despair (as all of us did). I never heard you curse your illness or your misfortune (as all of us did). I loved your patience, your willingness to wait and hope. Although we never disclosed to you the seriousness and finality of your illness, your superb intelligence must certainly long ago have led you to that conclusion, but you never collapsed nor yielded your hope and your faith.

On Sundays, I remember so vividly how you would literally totter to the altar rail to receive Holy Communion. You would come back to the pew, bow your head, and, I imagine, would ask for help and guidance from Jesus Christ, whom you knew and loved. Chris, you had found God, I'm sure, and I will try to find Him once again. I love you, Chris.

YOUR DAD

FROM MARK:

As mentioned in the book, I was raised as a Roman Catholic. For many years I went through the various rituals: first confession and communion, confraternity classes and confirmation. Yet, God was not real to me. Chris became sick and I still went to church every Sunday. I prayed. As time went on Chris grew worse. Eventually, my faith dwindled. I loved him, and to see a boy just coming into manhood suffer physical and mental anguish went through me like a sharp sword.

For quite a while during my high school years, I played in a rock and roll band. We were rather a rowdy bunch. After a few years, we broke up and eventually graduated and went our separate ways.

About two years after graduation, I ran into the bass player from the band, Joel, a boisterous guy when I knew him before. Now something was radically different about him. He started telling me about the love of Jesus Christ. I was astonished! He had really changed. This wasn't like the old Joel. When we were in the band together, he used to ridicule me and make me look foolish. Now, he was asking me about my spiritual life and he really cared.

About this time Chris was laid up in bed and was very weak. Joel was praying for me and having his friends pray for me. He was also attending the local Peninsula Baptist Church and asked me on occasion to come with him. I consented. I saw something at this church and in Joel that I had never seen before in any other church; love and concern, not insofar as particular denominations are concerned, but that Jesus Christ is a daily experience in our lives. Chris died but Joel kept coming around and sharing with me.

I didn't realize it then, but I know now that Chris' death was a plan of God. Two things have happened to me: First, my brother and I have become much closer. Second, not until sometime quite later did I become a real Christian. Through Chris' death, the Lord had many blessings for me. He comforted me greatly and I believe the Lord will use this experience to help me relate to others who have gone through the same situation. The Lord is real in my life. To those people who question the existence of God, my answer is an unconditional "yes."

MARK

FROM KEVIN:

It doesn't seem possible that it has been almost two years since Chris' death. When I reflect on his death now, the same sense of disbelief and confusion I felt right after he passed away comes back to me. The horror is a thing of the past now, but I wonder if I will ever be able to realize and accept it as a natural part of life.

My thoughts of him in his younger days and in the memory of his last four years, despite his illness, are happy and come to me often. I cannot begin to talk about these thoughts as they are things that only Chris and I could understand.

There are certain ways of relating, unspoken, mutual understandings during intimate and isolated moments in time, when two people who know each other very well and love each other very much are happy to share, and which no one else could ever quite appreciate.

These times and feelings between Chris and me are the ones that I remember. They are Chris' personal gifts to me. I will always hold them close and treasure them. Living through Chris' death has influenced much of my thinking about life, the world, and religion. The questions about God which imposed themselves so heavily during the period of Chris' illness are of little importance to me now. What is important is living a good and full life, loving those around me, and appreciating each moment of my life as completely as possible. There is no reason to chastise or plead with, or pray to a God who we do not even know exists. If there is a God, he is, by definition, beyond chastisement. He is perfect. If we do not know that there is a God, a more honest expression than prayer would be to share love for each other and a sincere reverence for life in everything we do. We would be relating to things we know are real. Living in a good and honest way with the world around us, with those things that we see and feel and know exist, is the best that any of us can do.

There are many things in this world that we can learn about and experience. There is so much beauty to be absorbed and appreciated in nature ... so much to learn about the love in the people around me and the people I will meet in the future, and so much to find out about myself. There is so little time. I have more than I will ever be able to look at in the world around me. I do not need to look for anything else outside of this world.

If I should ever find a God, that would be good. But, meanwhile, there are other things that have a much greater claim on my time and energy.

These are things that come to my mind when I think about what Chris' life meant to me. I hope that I will not forget the things that I have learned and the feelings that I have experienced as a result of knowing Chris.

KEVIN